Neural Interfaces

**IEEE Press**

445 Hoes Lane

Piscataway, NJ 08854

# Neural Interfaces

## Bridging Cognitive Neuroscience and Artificial Intelligence

*Avinash Singh*

*School of Computer Science and Australian AI Institute,*
*University of Technology Sydney, Australia*

IEEE Press
WILEY

Published by John Wiley & Sons, Inc., Hoboken, New Jersey.



***Library of Congress Cataloging-in-Publication Data***

Names: Singh, Avinash (Of University of Technology, Sydney) author
Title: Neural interfaces : bridging cognitive neuroscience and artificial intelligence / Avinash Singh.
Description: Hoboken, New Jersey : John Wiley & Sons, Inc, [2026] | Includes bibliographical references.
Identifiers: LCCN 2026016620 | ISBN 9781394331819 hardback | ISBN 9781394331833 adobe pdf | ISBN 9781394331826 epub | ISBN 9781394331840 ebook
Subjects: LCSH: Brain-computer interfaces | Cognitive neuroscience | Artificial intelligence
Classification: LCC QP360.7 .S55 2026
LC record available at https://lccn.loc.gov/2026016620

Cover Design: Wiley
Cover Image: Who is Danny/stock.adobe.com

*To my family*

# Contents

## About the Author

**Dr Avinash Singh** is a Senior Lecturer at the School of Computer Science, University of Technology Sydney (UTS), and Director of the Human Augmentation Lab. His work focuses on advancing brain–computer interfaces (BCIs), neuroadaptive systems, human augmentation, and technologies for enhancing human cognition in real-world settings. His research sits at the intersection of machine learning, cognitive neuroscience, and mixed reality, with a particular emphasis on building robust two-way BCI systems that enhance cognition, support decision-making, and improve everyday human–technology interactions.

Dr Singh is also actively involved in global conversations around neurotechnology ethics, standards, and research practices. He serves as an Editorial Member for *Scientific Reports* (Nature Portfolio) and as an Academic Editor for *PLOS Digital Health*. He also serves as Co-Chair of the IEEE Neuroethics Framework for the Workplace, with support from IEEE Brain, is a member of the IEEE Standards Committee on Unifying Brain–Computer Interfaces, contributes as an Expert Advisory Panel member for The Centre for Neurotechnology and Law (CNL), founding executive council member for CNL ANZ chapter, and works with UNICEF as an Expert Advisor for the *Neurotechnology for Children* initiative. He received the Google TensorFlow Faculty Award in 2021 and founded the India Future Society.

He earned his PhD from UTS in 2019, collaborating with institutions in Germany and the US, and holds a Master's degree from BITS Pilani, completed in 2013.

# Preface

Brain–computer interfaces (BCIs) have always been attractive to scientists, clinicians, technologists, hobbyists, and writers. BCI had begun as an effort to help people with severe paralysis that allow them to communicate and regain a sense of agency but since then expanded into a broader exploration of how the human mind can interact with machines. In the last 50 years, the field has significant progresses and advances in cognitive neuroscience together with recent developments in artificial intelligence (AI) and machine learning have sparked a renewed momentum in the field of BCI. This book is written to offer a clear and integrated perspective on this rapidly evolving landscape. I have tried not to make the focus of this book solely on technical methods or clinical applications, but my aim is to bridge the gap between foundational cognitive neuroscience knowledge and recent AI techniques, together with the real-world challenges in creating BCIs. My goal is to provide readers with both the basic understanding of BCI, its foundation in cognitive neuroscience, and how and why BCIs are developed, tested, and ultimately translated into applications. As BCIs move beyond controlled laboratory settings to everyday environments, they carry the potential to redefine interaction, accessibility, and, importantly, personal agency. It also raises questions around ethics, privacy, and how human will work with machines and with each other in the future. This book is intended as an introductory guide through this complex terrain, offering ideas from research, industry, and existing practices to help readers navigate the opportunities and responsibilities that accompany such transformative and disruptive technology. I hope that reading this book inspires curiosity and encourages thoughtful conversation about the field. The future of BCI is very exciting, and I hope you will join me in this exciting journey.

Sydney
Nov 2025

# Acknowledgments

The invitation to write this book was an exciting and unforgettable moment for me and perhaps a milestone for me as an academic and researcher. As a first-time sole author for book, the idea of transforming my experience in the field of BCI, all the thoughts, readings, curiosity, and aspirations poured into book was so exciting and overwhelming. However, make no mistake, writing a book is a mammoth task and I have even more respect for writers ever before. Book writing task needs a strict discipline, clarity, and countless hours of reflection and as always art of storytelling. I began this project with so many ideas however over time I realized that I could not fit them all in one book, and it may read weird if I did. I left those ideas for future book writing assignment if I get another opportunity. To be realistic and stay within the timeline, I had to prioritize, filter, and reshape these ideas many times into what I believe is the most meaningful and accessible version for readers. I have completed major part of writing during my extended annual leave from academic job which allowed me to dedicate myself fully and make major progress on the core sections and chapters of the book. I am very grateful to my family and friends to continuous support throughout this writing process. To my friends, I extend my sincere thanks for their encouragement and energy to me whenever the work felt too heavy. Above all, I am very thankful to my wife because she patiently provided my all the love and steady belief I need during this entire effort. Their support allowed me to go from first page to the last. In addition to thanking humans, I do want to thank a significant progress in AI, particularly LLMs, which also allowed me interesting discussion with my ideas that have shaped this book as well. I would also like to express my sincere appreciation to my publisher, Wiley, for their continued support and understanding throughout the process. Their flexibility, including several extensions on deadlines and several requests, made it possible for me to shape this book with the care and attention it required. Finally, I would like to thank you, the reader. It is my hope that this book will spark your curiosity and encourage you to explore further the exciting and rapidly evolving world of neural interfaces and brain-computer interface with amazing future possibilities.

Avinash Singh

# Acronyms

| | |
|---|---|
| **A1** | Primary Auditory Cortex |
| **ACC** | Anterior Cingulate Cortex |
| **aDBS** | Adaptive Deep Brain Stimulation |
| **AE** | Autoencoder |
| **AEP** | Auditory Evoked Potential |
| **AGI** | Artificial General Intelligence |
| **AI** | Artificial Intelligence |
| **ALPHA** | Alpha Band (8–12 Hz) |
| **AMY** | Amygdala |
| **ANN** | Artificial Neural Network |
| **API** | Application Programming Interface |
| **AR** | Augmented Reality |
| **ATTN** | Attention Mechanism |
| **AUC** | Area Under the Curve |
| **Autoreject** | Automated Artifact Rejection Tool (Python) |
| **BCI** | Brain-computer Interface |
| **BCIlab** | MATLAB-based BCI Development Framework |
| **BETA** | Beta Band (13–30 Hz) |
| **BIDS** | Brain Imaging Data Structure |
| **BMI** | Brain-machine Interface |
| **BOLD** | Blood Oxygen Level Dependent Signal |
| **Braindecode** | Deep Learning Toolbox for EEG/ECoG |
| **BrainFlow** | Cross-platform EEG/BCI Data Acquisition Framework |
| **cGAN** | Conditional Generative Adversarial Network |
| **CLI** | Command Line Interface |
| **CNN** | Convolutional Neural Network |
| **CPU** | Central Processing Unit |
| **CWT** | Continuous Wavelet Transform |

| | |
|---|---|
| **DARPA** | Defense Advanced Research Projects Agency |
| **DBS** | Deep Brain Stimulation |
| **DC** | Direct Current Signal |
| **DE** | Differential Entropy |
| **Deep1010** | Standardized EEG Channel Ordering for Deep Learning |
| **Deep4Net** | Deep4Net Architecture |
| **DELTA** | Delta Band (0.5–4 Hz) |
| **DL** | Deep Learning |
| **DLPFC** | Dorsolateral Prefrontal Cortex |
| **DMN** | Default Mode Network |
| **DoD** | Department of Defense |
| **DRY** | Dry Electrodes |
| **DWT** | Discrete Wavelet Transform |
| **ECoG** | Electrocorticography |
| **EEG** | Electroencephalography |
| **EEGLAB** | MATLAB Toolbox for EEG Analysis |
| **EEGNet** | EEGNet Deep Learning Architecture |
| **EHR** | Electronic Health Record |
| **ELBO** | Evidence Lower Bound |
| **EMG** | Electromyography |
| **EMR** | Electronic Medical Record |
| **EMS** | Electrical Muscle Stimulation |
| **ERD** | Event-related Desynchronization |
| **ERP** | Event-related Potential |
| **ErrP** | Error-related Potential |
| **ERS** | Event-related Synchronization |
| **FCM** | Fuzzy C-means Clustering |
| **FD** | Fractal Dimension |
| **FDA** | Food and Drug Administration |
| **FES** | Functional Electrical Stimulation |
| **FieldTrip** | MATLAB Toolbox for EEG/MEG/ECoG Analysis |
| **fMRI** | Functional Magnetic Resonance Imaging |
| **fNIRS** | Functional Near-infrared Spectroscopy |
| **FPN** | Frontoparietal Network |
| **FRN** | Feedback-related Negativity |
| **fUS** | Functional Ultrasound Imaging |
| **GAMMA** | Gamma Band (30–100 Hz) |
| **GAN** | Generative Adversarial Network |
| **GCN** | Graph Convolutional Network |
| **GEL** | Gel-based Electrodes |
| **GMM** | Gaussian Mixture Model |

| | |
|---|---|
| **GPU** | Graphics Processing Unit |
| **GRU** | Gated Recurrent Unit |
| **GSR** | Galvanic Skin Response |
| **GUI** | Graphical User Interface |
| **hBCI** | Hybrid Brain-computer Interface |
| **HC** | Hippocampus |
| **HCI** | Human-computer Interaction |
| **HD-EEG** | High Density EEG |
| **HMM** | Hidden Markov Model |
| **HRV** | Heart Rate Variability |
| **ICA** | Independent Component Analysis |
| **IEEE** | Institute of Electrical and Electronics Engineers |
| **iEEG** | Intracranial Electroencephalography |
| **IFG** | Inferior Frontal Gyrus |
| **IPL** | Inferior Parietal Lobule |
| **ISA** | Independent Subspace Analysis |
| **IT** | Inferotemporal Cortex |
| **JSON** | JavaScript Object Notation |
| **KNN** | K-nearest Neighbors |
| **LDA** | Linear Discriminant Analysis |
| **LFP** | Local Field Potential |
| **LMA** | Linear Microelectrode Array |
| **LSL** | Lab Streaming Layer |
| **LSTM** | Long Short-term Memory Network |
| **LZC** | Lempel-Ziv Complexity |
| **M1** | Primary Motor Cortex |
| **MEA** | Microelectrode Array |
| **MEG** | Magnetoencephalography |
| **MI** | Motor Imagery |
| **MIT** | Massachusetts Institute of Technology |
| **ML** | Machine Learning |
| **MLP** | Multilayer Perceptron |
| **MNE** | MNE-python Neuroimaging Library |
| **MOABB** | Mother of All BCI Benchmarks |
| **mPFC** | Medial Prefrontal Cortex |
| **MRI** | Magnetic Resonance Imaging |
| **MSE** | Multiscale Entropy |
| **MT** | Middle Temporal Visual Area (V5) |
| **MU** | Mu Rhythm (8–13 Hz) |
| **N200** | Negative 200 ms Event-related Component |
| **NASA** | National Aeronautics and Space Administration |

| | |
|---|---|
| **NeuroKit2** | Physiological Signal Processing Library |
| **NFB** | Neurofeedback |
| **NIBIB** | National Institute of Biomedical Imaging and Bioengineering |
| **NIH** | National Institutes of Health |
| **NIRS** | Near-infrared Spectroscopy |
| **NumPy** | Numerical Python Library |
| **OFC** | Orbitofrontal Cortex |
| **OpenBCI** | OpenBCI Toolkit and Hardware Ecosystem |
| **OPM** | Optically Pumped Magnetometer |
| **OPM-MEG** | OPM-based Magnetoencephalography |
| **P300** | Positive 300 ms Event-related Component |
| **PCA** | Principal Component Analysis |
| **PCC** | Posterior Cingulate Cortex |
| **PE** | Permutation Entropy |
| **PFC** | Prefrontal Cortex |
| **PMC** | Premotor Cortex |
| **PPC** | Posterior Parietal Cortex |
| **PREP** | Preprocessing Pipeline for EEG Standardization |
| **PSD** | Power Spectral Density |
| **PyTorch** | Deep Learning Library |
| **QDA** | Quadratic Discriminant Analysis |
| **RAM** | Random Access Memory |
| **RL** | Reinforcement Learning |
| **RNN** | Recurrent Neural Network |
| **RNS** | Responsive Neurostimulation System |
| **ROC** | Receiver Operating Characteristic |
| **S1** | Primary Somatosensory Cortex |
| **scikit-learn** | Machine Learning Library for Python |
| **SciPy** | Scientific Python Library |
| **SCR** | Skin Conductance Response |
| **SDK** | Software Development Kit |
| **SEEG** | Stereoelectroencephalography |
| **ShallowFBCSPNet** | Shallow Filter-bank CSP Network |
| **SMA** | Supplementary Motor Area |
| **SNR** | Signal-to-noise Ratio |
| **SQUID** | Superconducting Quantum Interference Device |
| **SSVEP** | Steady-state Visually Evoked Potential |
| **SSxEP** | Steady-state Evoked Potential (vision/auditory/tactile) |
| **STFT** | Short-time Fourier Transform |

| | |
|---|---|
| **STG** | Superior Temporal Gyrus |
| **SVM** | Support Vector Machine |
| **TCN** | Temporal Convolutional Network |
| **tDCS** | Transcranial Direct Current Stimulation |
| **TensorFlow** | Deep Learning Framework |
| **TEP** | Tactile Evoked Potential |
| **TES** | Transcranial Electrical Stimulation |
| **THETA** | Theta Band (4–8 Hz) |
| **TMS** | Transcranial Magnetic Stimulation |
| **TorchEEG** | PyTorch Library for EEG Deep Learning |
| **TPJ** | Temporoparietal Junction |
| **TRF** | Transformer Model |
| **URL** | Uniform Resource Locator |
| **Utah** | Utah Microelectrode Array |
| **V1** | Primary Visual Cortex |
| **V2** | Secondary Visual Cortex |
| **V3** | Tertiary Visual Cortex |
| **V4** | Visual Area 4 |
| **V5** | Visual Motion Area / MT |
| **VAE** | Variational Autoencoder |
| **VEP** | Visual Evoked Potential |
| **ViT** | Vision Transformer |
| **vmPFC** | Ventromedial Prefrontal Cortex |
| **VR** | Virtual Reality |
| **WGAN** | Wasserstein GAN |
| **WT** | Wavelet Transform |
| **XFM** | Cross-modal Transformer |
| **XML** | Extensible Markup Language |
| **XR** | Extended Reality |

## About the Companion Website

This book is accompanied by a companion website.

**https://www.wiley.com/go/singh_bcneuroai**

To access the website materials, click on the link under Related Resources on the book's page on wiley.com. You can also find this by searching www.wiley.com for the ISBN 9781394331819.

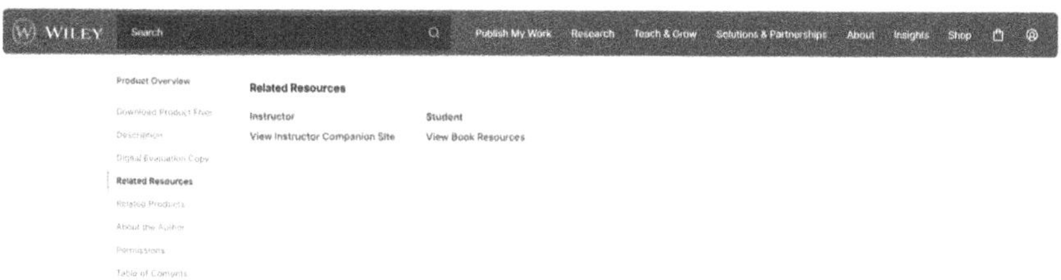


This website includes:

- Chapter-wise MCQs.

# Introduction

Neural interfaces encompass a broad class of technologies that record, decode, or stimulate neural activity to interact with the nervous system. These systems include neural prosthetics, neuromodulation devices, peripheral nerve interfaces, sensory restoration implants, and emerging bioelectronic medicines, but historically and in practice, the primary focus always has been on brain–computer interfaces (BCIs). Together, they represent a rapidly evolving field at the intersection of neuroscience, engineering, artificial intelligence, and human–machine interaction. Because of this central role, the evolution of BCIs provides an instructive lens through which to understand the development of neural interfaces as a whole. BCI technology was initially developed with the primary motivation of assisting individuals with quadriplegic paralysis. The goal was to provide a means for these individuals to interact with their surroundings through thought, such as controlling a wheelchair by imagining movements like left, right, forward, or backward. While BCI technology has largely remained stagnant over the last half-century, recent advancements in artificial intelligence (AI) and significant efforts from researchers and industry are transforming the landscape. In the next five years, BCI will see a significant transition from primarily traditional lab-based and experimental applications to more real-world and consumer-oriented solutions. BCI will evolve beyond conventional approaches, such as imagining motor movements, to become highly natural and hyper-personalized interfaces.

As a highly interdisciplinary field, BCI will affect the interaction of all existing digital technology, learning tools, training modules, self-monitoring and diagnosis systems, and mental health treatments. The extensive data collected through BCIs will significantly enhance our understanding of neuroscience and further refine and fuel the development of advanced AI algorithms, driving advancements across multiple domains.

"Neural Interface: Bridging Cognitive Neuroscience and Artificial Intelligence" offers new insights from an interdisciplinary angle into cognitive neuroscience and artificial intelligence to create sophisticated BCIs. This book explores and informs on how fundamental cognitive neuroscience knowledge takes shape into real-world BCI applications, going through the journey from experimentation to implementation. This book also delves into the technical understanding of mobile experimentation, machine learning, and tools and technology that are accelerating the development of BCIs, which may impact a significant number of people and potentially fundamentally change how we interact. The book covers a wide array of topics, including:

Historical Evolution of BCIs: This chapter explores the first neural experiments about 100 years ago to cutting-edge advancements and discover the key milestones that have shaped the BCI field. This chapter also highlights different BCI technologies available today and their effectiveness.

Fundamentals of Cognitive Neuroscience: Delves into fundamental understanding of the brain's structure and cognitive functioning, particularly of interest from BCI.

Neuroimaging Techniques and Applications: Learn about the tools and techniques in the research community for BCI applications focused on noninvasive techniques.

AI in Neural Interfaces: Explore how AI and machine learning are transforming the capabilities of BCIs. Explore the methods to decode neural signals and translate them into actionable commands. This chapter further talks about role of current generative AI in BCI.

Neuroethics: Given the potential and future impact of BCI technology, this chapter highlights the importance of developing such a technology responsibly with ethical considerations and implications of interfacing with the human brain. This chapter discusses the current perception from society and case studies.

Translational Neuroscience: Understand the process of turning research into real-world applications both in public and industries.

Experiment Paradigms and Tools: Learn about the experimental setups and tools crucial for BCI research.

Multimodality in BCIs: Explore the integration of multiple sensory inputs to enhance BCI functionality with examples and case studies. BCI Applications: This chapter provides a detailed example of application of BCI in three major stakeholder – Medical, which is the major motivation of BCI technology, Entertainment and Industry/Workplace. This chapter explores how BCIs are being used to restore lost functions, from neuroprosthetics to rehabilitation, diagnose mental disorders, augment psychological functions and used to improve performance.

Enhancing Human Capabilities: Investigate how BCIs can augment human abilities and expand the potential to achieve natural BCIs beyond traditionally known BCIs. Future of Brain–Computer Interfaces: Look ahead at the innovations and challenges that will shape the future of BCIs.

**Brain, Wires, and Waves**

The cortex is a system active every hour of the day,
Its networks fire in rhythms theta to gamma waves at play.
Who am I to judge a structure built of coded parts,
When consciousness itself emerges from its neural arts?

To study its design, we place our sensors with care,
Mapping signals as they synchronize with stimuli in air.
We transform the world through sensors that sync,
Turning data into meaning through each cortical design.

Brain-to-brain communication rises from decoding the mind,
A freedom shaped by models that track the will's design.
The brain centralize where computations gain dimension,
And AI joins the process extending human intention.

# 1

# Origins, Evolution, and Inspiration

The aspiration to have a direct communication pathway between the brain and external devices has always attracted researchers and scientists. Brain-computer interfaces (BCIs) aims to realize this vision by restoring motor function in patients with neurological disorders, enhancing cognitive performance, cognitive monitoring, as well as perhaps new forms of human-machine interaction. Over the last decades, both invasive and noninvasive methods to acquire brain signals have been improved. On one side, invasive methods require implanting electrodes into or onto neural tissues, while on the other side, noninvasive methods enable brain signals directly from the scalp using electroencephalography (EEG). Early experiments on recording and processing brain signals laid the groundwork for the modern BCIs. These methods are still applicable and essentially precursors of today's progress in cutting-edge BCIs. The evolution of technology, as shown in Figure 1.1 from simple amplifiers and oscilloscopes to high-density microelectrode arrays and advanced machine learning (ML) algorithms, has transformed BCIs from early theoretical constructs to practical devices.

## 1.1 Conceptual Foundations Before BCI

### 1.1.1 Early Fiction and Philosophy of Mind–Machine Interaction

Although the term BCI did not exist in the 18th and 19th century and no functional BCI technologies were present, both fiction and nonfiction literature from the era began exploring ideas that conceptually align with BCIs as we know now. Themes such as mental control by machines, artificial intelligence (AI), and human–machine integration were touched upon in early works. In *Illustrations of Madness* (1810), John Haslam documents a patient experiencing delusions of

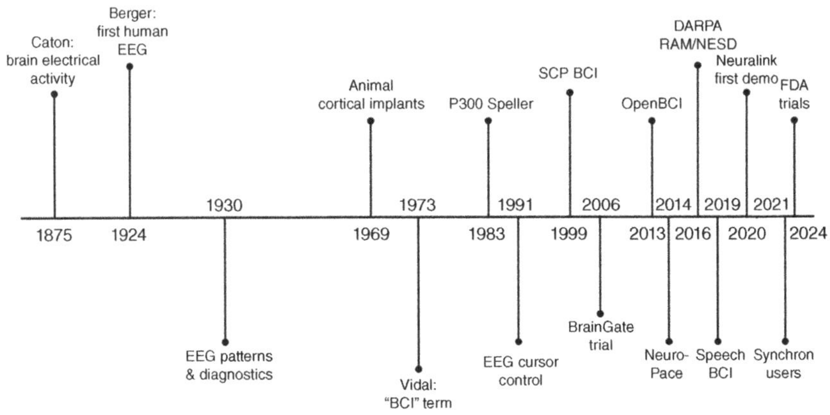


**Figure 1.1** A timeline in the development of different kind of neural interfaces.

an "influencing machine" that controlled his thoughts, arguably one of the earliest references to the concept of external devices affecting the mind [1]. Samuel Butler's *Erewhon* (1872) speculated on self-awareness and the evolution of machines, which indirectly encouraged debates around artificial cognition and autonomy [2]. In the French novel *The Future Eve* (1886), Villiers de l'Isle-Adam introduces an artificial android named Hadaly, exploring the emotional relationship between human and machine [3].

In the 20th-century fiction, BCI like ideas appeared frequently in works. In Frank Herbert's *Dune* (1965), an abstract form of cognitive augmentation is shown, which is used for training human computers called Mentats [4]. In Robert A. Heinlein's *The Moon Is a Harsh Mistress* (1966), a sentient computer is also featured interacting closely with humans in some kind of computer interface, similar to the idea of a brain-machine interface [5]. Michael Crichton's *The Terminal Man* (1972) also shows a character with a neural implant to control seizures, raising early concerns around brain control [6], similar to modern-world ethical issues. Then there is William Gibson's *Johnny Mnemonic* (1981), in which data couriers directly store information in their brains, another example of brain-machine integration [7]. Gibson's *Neuromancer* (1984) further extends his idea and writes on a cyberpunk future, where characters "Jack" interface with cyberspace via neural implants [8]. Finally, Masamune Shirow's *Ghost in the Shell* (1989) stands out as a cyberpunk manga in which cybernetic humans interface directly with networks via BCIs, exploring themes of identity, consciousness, and what it means to possess a "ghost" (soul) within a machine body [9]. Figure 1.2 shows one of the panels from this manga where a robot and a human brain are interfacing. These early works laid the imaginative groundwork for later BCI narratives.

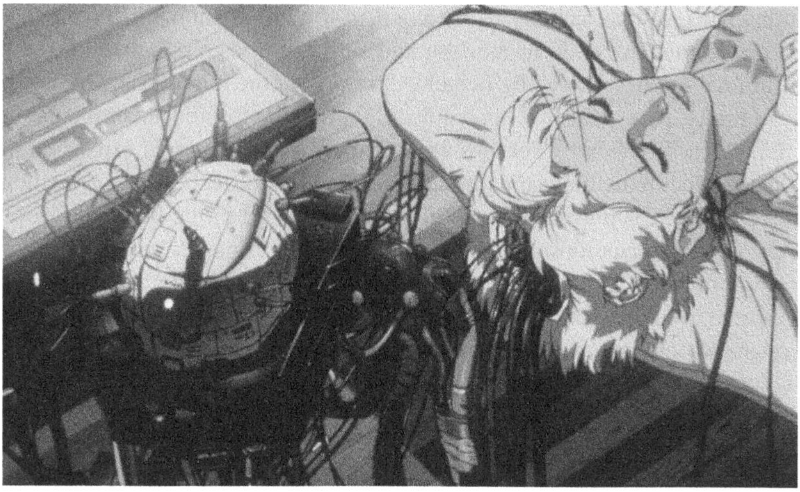

Moviestore Collection Ltd / Alamy Stock Photos

**Figure 1.2** Picture from *Ghost in the Shell* by Masamune Shirow.

### 1.1.2 18th–19th Century Electrophysiology

The conceptual origin of BCI technology can be traced back to all the foundational work that happened in the 18th and 19th centuries. One of the earliest works accredited to Italian physiologist Luigi Galvan, who explored the electrical nature of biological systems. He demonstrated in the 1780s that frog muscles twitch in response to electrical stimulation and called it "animal electricity" [10]. This laid the groundwork for understanding the nervous system as an electrically active medium. Building on this foundation, German scientist Emil du Bois-Reymond expanded the study of bioelectricity in the mid-1800s, successfully measuring the electrical impulses of nerves and muscles and describing what would later be known as action potentials [11]. Later, in 1875, British physician Richard Caton showed in an experiment the first ever spontaneous electrical activity in the exposed brains of living animals and measured cortical potential using a galvanometer [12]. Although these works are not directly related to BCI, they have provided a deeper physiological understanding and experimental basis which is still applicable and the basis of most modern BCI devices.

## 1.2 Scientific Milestones of the 20th Century

### 1.2.1 Discovery of Cortical Signals (1900s–1950s)

The conceptual foundations of interfacing between brain and machine can be traced back to early experiments in electrophysiology and neurophysiology. During the early 1900s, researchers such as Richard Caton and Hans Berger began exploring the electrical activity of the brain in the lab as shown in Figure 1.3. Caton's continuous work from the 19th and 20th centuries on electrical activity in the animal brain, followed by Berger's discovery of the human EEG noninvasively in the 1920s, established the empirical foundation for understanding brain function [13, 14]. The early decades were characterized by a rapid expansion of knowledge in neuroanatomy and physiology. Although the technology of the time did not permit the sophisticated recordings later realized in the BCI field. However, theoretical discussions and initial experimental techniques set the stage for later developments. For instance, the demonstration that electrical signals could be measured from the scalp was revolutionary, paving the way for the concept that brain signals could be harnessed for external applications.

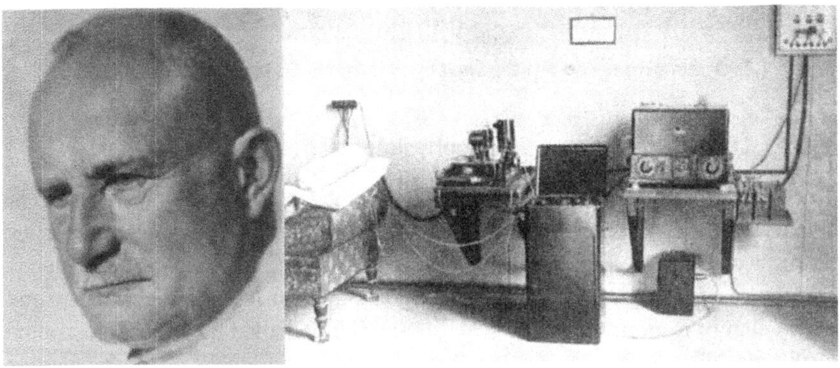

(a)

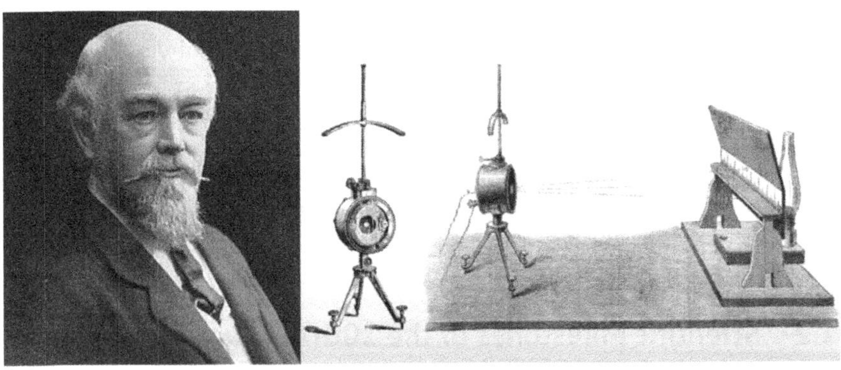

(b)

**Figure 1.3** (a) Hans Berger and (b) Richard Caton and their experimentation system.

### 1.2.2 From Observation to Interaction

The period following World War II between the 1950s and 1970s saw significant advances in electronics and signal processing, which accelerated the development of research in the direction of BCI. The emergence of the transistor and later integrated circuits provided researchers with tools for better amplifying and processing the weak neural signals that had been observed in earlier decades [15]. This era witnessed a growing interest in using neural signals and harness them, although the term "BCI" was not coined yet.

Researchers began conceptualizing experiments on how to modulate EEG rhythms. Early studies by Jacques Vidal at University of California, Los Angeles (UCLA), start exploring the possibilities and feasibility of an EEG-based communication system and are now seen as pioneering efforts that laid the groundwork [17]. Although these studies were limited by the available technology, they underscored the potential of brain signals as a medium for direct communication with machines. During this period, invasive methods are starting to attract researchers. Animal studies employing direct cortical recordings revealed that specific patterns of neural activity could be correlated with movement intentions. Although the clinical translation of these findings was still far off, these experiments were critical in demonstrating that invasive recordings could provide high-resolution insights into brain function [16].

### 1.2.3 Birth of BCI Field

Modern BCI research began in the 1970s with Jacques Vidal's pioneering work on direct brain-to-computer communication, with setups as big as the large room shown in Figure 1.4 and the first ever introduction of the term "BCI" in his 1973 publication [17]. His early experiments were based on EEG to detect neural signals and translate them into simple commands, primarily for motor control and communication. As research progressed in the following decade after Vidal's work, advancements in signal processing, ML, and neural decoding further expanded BCI capabilities. There was significant progress in the 1990s, especially in non-invasive EEG-based BCI systems, including pioneering work on the P300-speller in 1988 [18] and the foundation of the motor imagery BCI paradigm in 1994 [19].

After Vidal's work, another significant progress was made in the seminal work by Niels Birbaumer [20] in 1999, where he demonstrated a slow cortical potential-based BCI that allowed locked-in patients to communicate. This was a significant breakthrough in the world of BCI to assist individuals with severe motor impairments. He showed that a patient with a brain implant is able to spell out words in German, as shown in Figure 1.5.

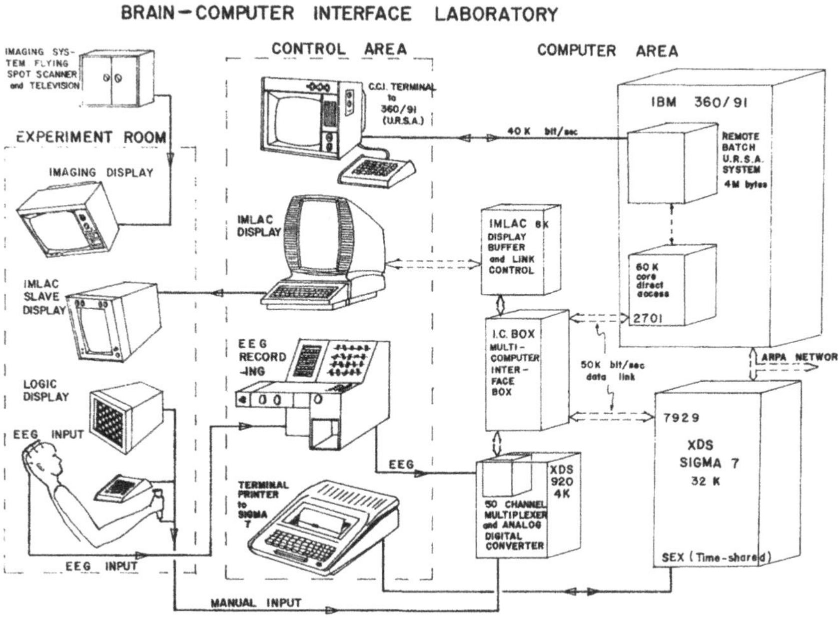


**Figure 1.4** Vidal BCI setup in UCLA which is known as BCI laboratory. *Source*: [17]/with permission of Annual Reviews.

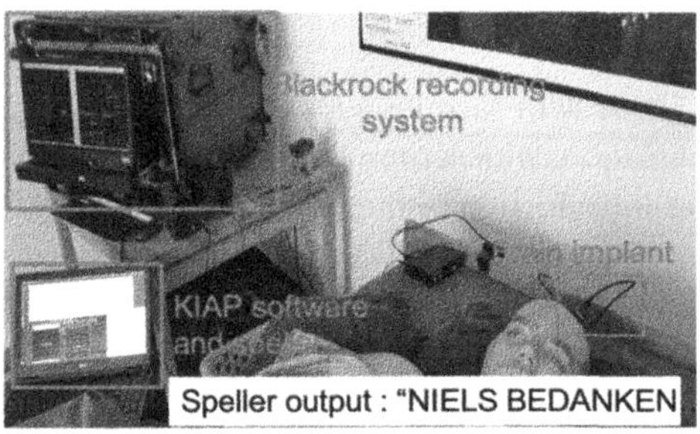


**Figure 1.5** One of first BCI system where patient is able to write a message through brain signals taken. *Source*: [21]/Springer Nature/CC BY 4.0.

### 1.2.4 Key Developments in Modern BCI

The early 2000s marked a significant turning point in BCI research, with a shift from conceptual demonstrations to clinical applications. One of the most notable breakthroughs was the development of the BrainGate system [22], which utilized intracortical electrodes to allow individuals with severe motor disabilities to control external devices such as robotic arms and computer cursors. These works have provided clear evidence toward enabling communication and motor functionality by decoding high-resolution brain signals. From 2010 onward, the BCI field has seen a rapid upward trajectory in terms of progress and innovation, probably due to initiatives like the Defence Advanced Research Projects Agency (DARPA), Neuralink, and Synchron. They are pushing boundaries to make BCI wireless, with high density of electrodes, miniaturized implants, and long-term usability. Though detailed discussions on these advances are covered in later chapters, it is worth noting that this period has also been characterized by increasing clinical translation, with human trials expanding in scope and scale. Simultaneously, consumer interest in noninvasive BCIs has grown, leading to the development of portable EEG headsets, open-source platforms, and BCI applications in gaming and wellness. These developments have broadened the scope of BCI research beyond clinical contexts, creating a dynamic and multidisciplinary ecosystem.

See Table 1.1 for a summary of key developments in BCIs, from early fiction to foundational electrophysiology and 20th-century experiments contributing to growing interest and application of BCIs.

**Table 1.1** BCI history timeline.

| Year | Milestone | Description |
|---|---|---|
| **1875** [13] | Richard Caton discovers brain electrical activity | First evidence of electrical signals in the brain via animal studies |
| **1924** [14] | Hans Berger records first human EEG | Inventor of electroencephalography (EEG); foundation of noninvasive BCI |
| **1930s–1950s** | EEG further developed for medical diagnostics | Recognized patterns (e.g., alpha, beta waves); used in epilepsy, sleep research |
| **1960s [23, 24]** | First animal neurophysiology recordings with implants | Implanted electrodes used in cats and monkeys for motor and visual cortex studies |
| **1970s** [17] | J.J. Vidal coins term BCI and builds first system | First real-time BCI prototype; user could move cursor via EEG signals |
| **1980s [25]** | Direct cortical recording in monkeys | Advances in invasive BCI: understanding motor intention via neural spikes |
| **1988 [18]** | P300 Speller | First brain–computer interface enabling users to spell characters using the P300 detected by Electroencephalography |
| **1990 [26]** | Sensorimotor rhythm control | First evidence that users can voluntarily modulate Sensorimotor Rhythms to control a computer |

(*Continued*)

**Table 1.1** (Continued)

| Year | Milestone | Description |
|---|---|---|
| **1990s [22]** | BrainGate research begins (Brown University) | High-resolution invasive BCI research for motor control and communication |
| **2004** [27] | First BrainGate human trial | Paralyzed person controlled robotic arm via cortical implants |
| **2013** [28] | OpenBCI founded | Open-source, low-cost EEG BCI systems for research and experimentation |
| **2013** [29] | NeuroPaceFDA approval (responsive neurostimulation) | Closed-loop neural implant for epilepsy — early example of therapeutic BCI |
| **2013–2015** | DARPA invests heavily in BCI (RAM, NESD programs) | Focus on memory restoration, high-bandwidth brain communication |
| **2016** [30] | Neuralink founded by Elon Musk | Goal: high-bandwidth BCI with thousands of threads into the brain |
| **2019** [31] | First successful "speech BCI" using electrocorticography (ECoG) signals | Turned brain signals into synthetic speech in real time |
| **2020** [32] | Neuralink live demo (pig brain, wireless BCI) | Demonstrated real-time neural recording via coin-sized implant |
| **2021** [33] | First monkey plays Pong via Neuralink implant | Major media moment; showed functional motor decoding |
| **2023** [34] | Blackrock Neurotech and Synchron report long-term users | Real-world trials of BCIs for paralyzed patients controlling tablets, typing |
| **2024–2025** [35] | FDA trials for human-grade implants (Neuralink, Synchron) | Focus on safety, telepathic communication, and real-time intention decoding |

## 1.3 Key Historical Milestones in Acquisition and Methods

### 1.3.1 Invasive BCIs

Invasive BCIs involve implanting electrodes directly into neural tissue, enabling high-fidelity recordings of neuronal activity. Although invasive methods pose greater risks and technical challenges, they have the advantage of capturing detailed spatiotemporal patterns of neural firing that are often obscured by the filtering effects of noninvasive techniques.

#### 1.3.1.1 Neural Recording Techniques and Early Invasive Studies

Early invasive BCI studies primarily focused on animal models. In the 1960s and 1970s, researchers demonstrated that individual neurons or small populations of neurons in the motor cortex could be recorded using microelectrodes. Seminal work by Evarts [36] and others provided evidence that neurons in the motor cortex exhibited activity patterns related to limb movement. These studies laid the foundation for subsequent developments in neural decoding, whereby the intended movements of an organism could be inferred from neural activity. Specially, the work of Georgopoulos in the 1980s has demonstrated that the direction of intended motor movement could be decoded from the specific firing patterns of a population of neurons [37]. These findings help researchers in better understanding of motor control but also provided a foundational basis for developing BCI systems for controlling prosthetic limbs from brain signals.

#### 1.3.1.2 Developments in Implantable Electrodes and Microelectrode Arrays

The development of implantable microelectrode arrays marked a significant milestone in invasive BCI research. Arrays such as the Utah array, introduced in the 1990s, enabled simultaneous recording from hundreds of neurons, thus greatly enhancing the spatial resolution of neural recordings [38]. This technology provided a robust platform for studying the fine structure of neural representations of movement and for developing decoding algorithms that could translate neural activity into control commands for external devices. One of the most influential studies in this domain was conducted by Schwartz and colleagues, who used multielectrode recordings to control robotic arms in primates (Figure 1.6) [39]. This work demonstrated the feasibility of real-time decoding of neural signals and provided an experimental framework that spurred subsequent research in the field. In parallel, researchers were also developing implantable stimulation devices, paving the way for bidirectional BCIs that could both read from and write to neural circuits [40].

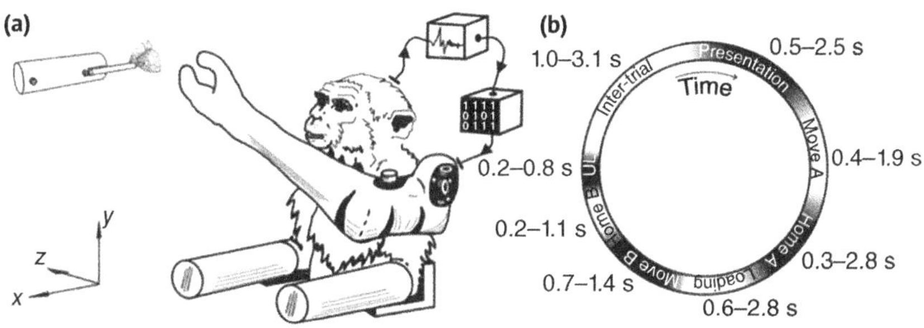


**Figure 1.6** Monkey is controlling a prosthetic arm for self-feeding. *Source:* [39]/with permission of Springer Nature.

#### 1.3.1.3 Clinical Applications and Long-term Implant Studies

The use of invasive BCI technologies for clinical application has started in the late 1990s and early 2000s. These applications were based on individuals who had severe motor impairments such as amyotrophic lateral sclerosis (ALS) or spinal cord injury and provided early evidence in the efficacy of invasive BCIs to support communication and control capabilities [20]. Hochberg et al. [28] show in a landmark study that invasive BCI can allow patients with tetraplegia to control a cursor using neural activity. Long-term implant studies have provided insights into the stability and reliability of chronic neural recordings. These studies highlight the challenges associated with electrode degradation, immune response, and the need for adaptive decoding algorithms that can compensate for shifts in neural signal properties over time. Despite these challenges, the success of invasive BCIs in clinical settings has motivated continued research into improving biocompatibility and signal quality.

### 1.3.2 Noninvasive Brain–Computer Interfaces

Noninvasive BCIs, most commonly based on EEG and functional near-infrared spectroscopy (fNIRS), offer the significant advantage of lower risk and easier implementation. However, they also present challenges such as lower spatial resolution and susceptibility to noise. This section looks at the evolution of noninvasive BCI technologies and their applications.

#### 1.3.2.1 Electroencephalography-based BCIs

EEG-based BCIs are known as noninvasive BCI systems that can measure electrical potentials from brain activity from the scalp. In 1990, Wolpaw demonstrated that individuals could learn to control EEG rhythms related to motor control and use them to control external devices [41]. These exciting outputs fuel the progress in the field. Over the past two decades, EEG-based BCI systems have grown significantly due to advances in signal processing along with the success of techniques such as common spatial patterns (CSP) [42], independent component analysis (ICA) [43], and now deep learning models [44]. Currently, EEG can be seen in a variety of BCI applications ranging from cursor control, spelling devices, to controlling prosthetic limbs and exoskeletons.

A significant milestone in EEG-BCI research was the development of the P300 speller paradigm [45]. This paradigm is based on event-related potentials (ERPs) to enable communication for locked-in patients. The P300 speller has been extensively validated and remains one of the most successful noninvasive BCI applications to date. Despite challenges such as signal variability and susceptibility to artifacts, EEG continues to be a essential in BCI research due to its noninvasive nature and ease of use.

#### 1.3.2.2 Functional Magnetic Resonance Imaging (fMRI) and Near-infrared Spectroscopy (NIRS)

Beyond EEG, other noninvasive imaging modalities have been explored for BCI applications. Functional magnetic resonance imaging (fMRI) provides high spatial resolution images of brain activity, albeit with lower temporal resolution compared to EEG. They were introduced to BCI research in the late 1990s. Early studies using fMRI-based BCIs demonstrated that participants could learn to control certain aspects of brain activity, however within the confines of an MRI scanner [46]. While fMRI-BCIs have offered unique insights into the spatial dynamics of brain activity, however, their practical applications have been limited due to the cost, complexity, and immobility of MRI systems.

Near-infrared spectroscopy (NIRS) has also emerged as an alternative noninvasive modality, with initial BCI applications beginning in the early 2000s. NIRS measures changes in blood oxygenation and has been applied to BCI tasks, particularly in situations where EEG's sensitivity to artifacts is problematic [47]. Although the temporal resolution of NIRS is limited by the hemodynamic response, its ease of use and portability have made it attractive for certain applications, such as brain–computer gaming interfaces and simple control tasks.

#### 1.3.2.3 Emerging Noninvasive Modalities

There has been active exploration of alternate noninvasive techniques that can be used for BCIs. One such technique is magnetoencephalography (MEG), which measures the magnetic fields generated by neural activity. MEG can be seen as an alternative to EEG with potentially improved spatial resolution [48]. MEG is first applied to BCI research in the early 2000s. However, the need for specialized magnetically shielded environments has limited the widespread adoption of MEG-based BCIs. Another emerging modality is functional ultrasound (fUS) imaging, introduced to neuroimaging and BCI research in the mid-2010s, which has shown promise in preclinical studies for capturing neural dynamics with high spatial and temporal resolution [49]. Although still in the early stages of development for human applications, fUS may eventually complement existing noninvasive technologies by providing detailed maps of brain activity without the need for large and expensive equipment.

More detailed discussion on acquisition and stimulation technology is discussed in Chapter 3.

### 1.3.3 Signal Processing and ML in BCI Research

A key measure of invasive or noninvasive modalities for BCIs is whether it allows decoding neural signals that can be translatable into actionable commands. There has been significant progress in signal processing techniques since the early inception of BCI. These techniques have evolved from simple bandpass filtering and regression models to sophisticated ML algorithms to allow decoding complex neural signals. In some of the earliest BCI experiments 1970s and 1980s, the signal processing techniques were very basic, such as spectral analysis, bandpass filtering, and manual feature selection. These early research efforts used techniques like Fourier transforms and wavelet decompositions to extract signal features for simple binary tasks. By another decade in the 1990s and early 2000s, more systematic approaches to signal processing were developed for BCI. The introduction of ML marked a significant milestone for signal processing, and algorithms such as support vector machines (SVMs) and linear discriminant analysis (LDA) became standard tools for classifying neural patterns associated with specific motor intentions or cognitive states. These models provided better generalization across tasks and subjects compared to earlier rule-based approaches.

In the 2010s, the field experienced a major leap with the adoption of deep learning. Models such as convolutional neural networks (CNNs) and recurrent neural networks (RNNs) enabled automatic feature extraction directly from raw data, outperforming traditional models in decoding EEG signals [50]. These deep learning networks are very effective at capturing the spatiotemporal complexity of neural signals. In the late 2010s and into the 2020s, more advanced algorithms such as transfer learning and adaptive learning algorithms were introduced, which can solve issues like inter- and intra-subject variability, signal nonstationarity, and long-term usability. These techniques allow models to adapt over time to changes in the user's neural activity due to learning, fatigue, or electrode degradation, improving the robustness and longevity of BCI systems. As ML and AI techniques continue to evolve, the integration of transformer architectures and self-supervised learning with more accurate, flexible, and user-friendly BCIs continues to expand. This ongoing development and progress is reshaping how BCIs are designed, optimized, and personalized for real-world use. A detailed overview of signal processing and AI/ML is presented in Chapters 5 and 6.

### 1.3.4 Hybrid BCIs and Multimodal Interfaces

Hybrid BCIs combine two or more modalities to maximize the strengths and mitigate the weaknesses of individual techniques. Research into hybrid BCIs began to gain momentum in the late 2000s, as the limitations of single modality systems (particularly EEG) became more apparent. For example, combining EEG with fNIRS, a practice first explored around 2009–2010, can provide complementary information such as EEG offers high temporal resolution, while fNIRS contributes spatial resolution through hemodynamic signals. This multimodal approach has been shown to enhance the performance of BCIs in various tasks, ranging from simple cursor control to more complex decision-making processes [51].

Another promising direction in hybrid BCIs is the integration of invasive and noninvasive methods, a concept that began emerging in the early 2010s. In some cases, a noninvasive system can be used to augment or calibrate an invasive interface, leading to improved decoding accuracy and reduced calibration times. Similarly, hybrid systems also show improved performance of BCI by combining multiple that combine multiple noninvasive modalities such as EEG, MEG, and fNIRS. They have been developed since the mid-2010s to provide more robust and reliable control signals. To accommodate the diverse requirements of different applications, hybrid BCI systems are very useful. However, such hybrid systems also require complex signal processing and decoding processes that dynamically weight contributions of each modality and their performance. The versatility of hybrid systems, actively explored since the 2010s, lies in their ability to adapt to the specific constraints and goals of the task at hand.

The experimental studies in late 2010 have shown that hybrid BCIs are better in terms of accuracy, speed, and user satisfaction and outperform unimodal BCI systems. One of the key reasons behind this improvement is the complementary information between different modalities that allows for better prediction. In the future, with more research, hybrid BCIs could bridge the gap between experimental prototypes and market-ready BCI applications [52].

### 1.3.5 Ethical, Regulatory, and Societal Implications

BCI development is progressing rapidly; therefore, concerns related to the ethical use of this technology are also growing. There is increasing concern about BCI technology at the ethical, regulatory, and societal levels, and several discussions have taken place since the 2000s. Most of these discussions have particularly focused on invasive BCIs because they pose higher risks associated with surgical implantation, long-term biocompatibility issues, and the potential augmentation of neural functions [53]. Another factor contributing to these discussions is the significant progress made in invasive BCI experiments involving human participants during the 2000s. Moreover, the possibility of neural data being misused, whether for surveillance, manipulation, or other nefarious purposes, has led to a growing body of literature, especially from the mid-2010s onward, examining the ethical principles necessary to guide BCI research and deployment [54].

On the regulatory front, challenges began to emerge prominently in the late 2000s, as BCIs moved beyond research labs into clinical trials. The classification of BCIs as medical devices or consumer electronics has significant implications for the oversight of these systems. In many jurisdictions around the world, invasive BCIs are now subject to stringent clinical trial requirements and post-market surveillance to ensure safety and efficacy. Noninvasive BCIs, which gained consumer and therapeutic interest around the 2010s, are generally considered lower risk but still face regulatory issues related to data privacy, informed consent, and the standardization of performance metrics. Researchers and policymakers, particularly from the 2010s onward, have worked to develop guidelines that ensure the responsible development and deployment of BCI technologies.

The societal impact of BCIs extends beyond individual users to broader issues such as equity, accessibility, and social justice. These concerns became part of conversation more widely in the 2010s, as commercial interest in BCIs grew and applications for the general public became more feasible. Most of these concerns focus on the assumption that, if BCIs become widely available, they may create social inequalities because of their significant cost, which could place them out of reach for a large section of the population. At the same time, it is also true that BCIs hold significant potential to improve quality of life and personal autonomy for individuals with motor disabilities. Balancing these benefits and risks has become a central challenge for the field, especially in the 2020s as adoption accelerates. In addition, issues of informed consent and data security are significant, especially as BCIs slowing getting into daily life. The potential for "neurohacking" or unauthorized access to neural data is a real concern, which was first raised in academic circles in the early 2010s. That has prompted calls for robust cybersecurity measures and ethical oversight. As BCIs transition from experimental settings to widespread use, interdisciplinary collaborations among neuroscientists, engineers, ethicists, and legal experts have strengthened notably since the mid-2010s, and will be essential to ensure that these technologies are developed in a manner that is both innovative and socially responsible. More detail on this topic is discussed in Chapter 9.

## 1.4 Summary

The evolution of BCI we see today originated from ideas in literature and progressed through significant experiments in the early 20th century. Over the decades, a substantial number of interdisciplinary innovations have taken place. Both invasive and noninvasive BCIs have made significant advancements, each with its own challenges and applications. Invasive BCIs offer high spatiotemporal resolution and are therefore pivotal in enabling motor functions, whereas noninvasive BCIs, such as those based on EEG, support a range of applications from clinical to consumer-focused use.

Advances in signal processing and ML have been central to these developments, allowing researchers and developers to decode complex neural signals with increasing accuracy and reliability. Moreover, the emergence of hybrid and multimodal BCIs points to a future where the strengths of different modalities can be harnessed together to overcome individual limitations. While the technical achievements are impressive, the ethical, regulatory, and societal implications of

BCIs must be addressed as these technologies become more integrated into daily life. Although BCI technology has significant potential, it is equally important to ensure its safety, privacy, equitable access, and responsible development.

As BCI continues to develop, advances in sensor materials, ML, bidirectional interfaces, and emerging wearable concepts will drive new milestones in its evolution. These advances, coupled with rigorous ethical and regulatory frameworks, hold the promise of transforming our understanding of the brain, enhancing quality of life for individuals with disabilities, and creating unprecedented opportunities for human–machine interaction. As long as collaboration across disciplines continues to address BCI-related multifaceted challenges, it will continue to grow and play a transformative role in the future.

# 2

# Cognitive Neuroscience Foundations

A brain-computer interface (BCI) is a system that enables direct communication between the brain and an external device without needing to use neuromuscular pathways. Much of fundamental knowledge behind BCI systems is majorly attributed to cognitive neuroscience and relies on an understanding of measurable brain activities of several cognitive functions such as attention, perception, motor control, etc. The majority of these brain signals originate in the cerebral cortex where sensory processing, voluntary movement planning, and higher-order cognition take place. BCIs can infer user intent or mental states by decoding these cortical activities. Cortical activity is accessible both invasively and noninvasively and provide rich functional information. This functional information could be both active like motor imagery (MI) or passive such as attention, workload, stress, cognitive conflict, etc. However, modern cognitive neuroscience shows that subcortical structures also play an important role. Some examples such as the basal ganglia, thalamus, hippocampus, and limbic system shape behavior, learning, emotion, and decision-making. These deeper structures continuously interact with cortical circuits, therefore forming an integrated loop that essentially controls everything from habit formulation to affective regulation. As BCIs advance, insights from both cortical and subcortical systems are expanding the functional scope and adaptability of neural interfaces. Understanding how these brain regions contribute individually and cooperatively allows BCIs to move beyond simple motor control toward richer forms of communication, cognitive enhancement, and emotional or behavioral modulation. In the following sections, we explore how cortical and subcortical regions support and shape the capabilities of modern and future BCIs.

## 2.1 Brain Organization and Anatomy

To understand the foundations of cognitive neuroscience, It is important to understand how the brain is anatomically organized. This foundational understanding is essential for interpreting the neural signals used in BCI systems. The human brain is part of the nervous system, which is the body's communication and control system and allows it to receive information, process it, and send signals for the across body to move, feel, and respond. This nervous system can be divided into two major parts: the central nervous system (CNS) and the peripheral nervous system (PNS). The CNS includes the brain and spinal cord, which integrate sensory input, generate cognitive functions, and coordinate voluntary/involuntary actions (Figure 2.1). Whereas, the PNS connects the CNS to the rest of the body. The PNS can also be subdivided into the somatic nervous system (SNS) and the autonomic nervous system (ANS). The SNS is responsible for voluntary motor control and sensory transmission, whereas the ANS regulates involuntary physiological processes such as heart rate, digestion, and respiration. Within the CNS, the brain itself can be organized into two major functional domains highly relevant for BCIs: the *cortex* (or neocortex) and the *subcortical* structures (Figure 2.2). These two parts of the brain differ in evolutionary origin and structural complexity, yet they operate as an integrated system that shapes perception, thought, action, learning, and emotion.

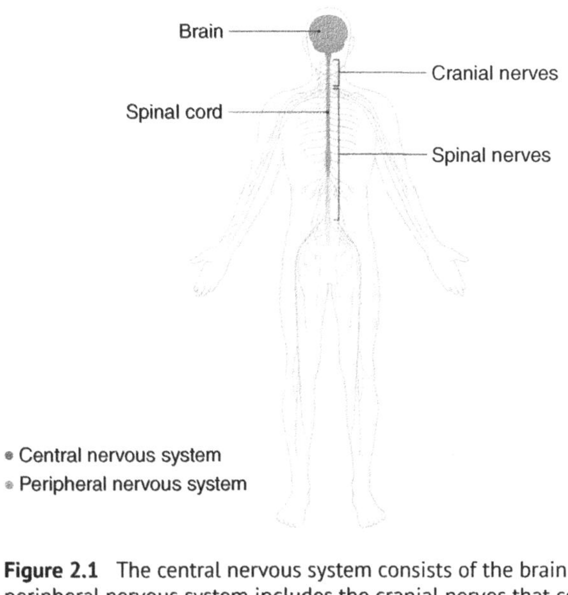


**Figure 2.1** The central nervous system consists of the brain and spinal cord, and the peripheral nervous system includes the cranial nerves that connect directly to the brain and the spinal nerves that connect to the spinal cord and extend throughout the rest of the body.

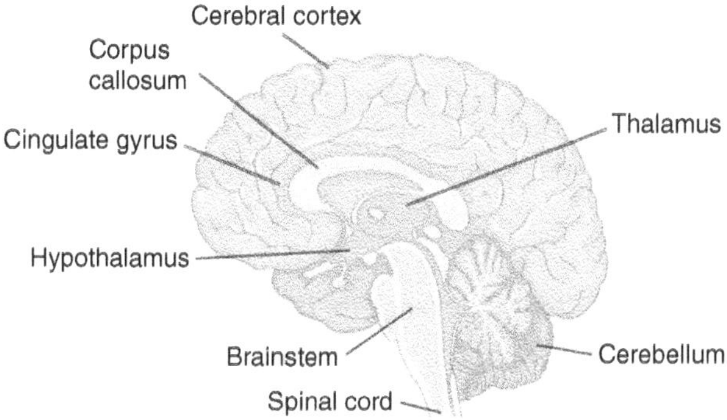


**Figure 2.2** Simplified anatomy of the human brain. The cerebral cortex is the outer folded layer of the brain. The corpus callosum bridges the left and right hemispheres. The thalamus controls sensory and motor information and hypothalamus helps regulate body temperature, hunger, thirst, sleep, and hormonal control. The brainstem connects the brain to the spinal cord and controls vital functions such as breathing and heart rate. The cerebellum supports coordination, balance, posture, and fine motor control. The spinal cord carries signals between the brain and the rest of the body.

### 2.1.1 The Cortex and Its Computational Architecture

The cerebral cortex is the evolutionarily newest part of the human brain and supports most of higher-order cognitive functions that BCIs attempt to decode in the current stage. Structurally, the cortex is a highly folded sheet of gray matter composed of billions of neurons arranged in distinct layers. This layered, columnar organization supports parallel processing, hierarchical connectivity, and large-scale integration of sensory, motor, and cognitive information. While later sections of this chapter describe the major cortical lobes and their BCI-relevant functions in detail, it is important to highlight two general properties:

#### 2.1.1.1 Functional Specialization

Different cortical regions support distinct computations such as motor planning, visual perception, language processing, or executive control that allow BCIs to target specific cognitive operations.

#### 2.1.1.2 Distributed Processing

Cortical functions emerge from interactions across widespread brain networks. This is essential to understand BCI signals that reflect coordinated neural dynamics.

Most of noninvasive brain signals, including electroencephalography (EEG), magnetoencephalography (MEG), and functional near-infrared spectroscopy (fNIRS), are based on cortical activities. Cortical activity produces large-scale electrical and hemodynamic signals which are accessible from the scalp. In contrast to noninvasive brain signals, invasive brain signals, including electrocorticography (ECoG) and intracortical arrays capture cortical circuit activity, which allows direct high-resolution signals for motor intentions, speech generation, sensory perception, and other functions.

### 2.1.2 Subcortical Systems and Their Relevance for BCI

Beneath the neocortex lie evolutionarily older subcortical structures that regulate motivation, emotion, reward learning, autonomic control, and the gating of actions. These structures include the thalamus, hypothalamus, basal ganglia, hippocampus, and amygdala, form interconnected loops with the cortex and exert modulatory effects on behavior. Subcortical regions are increasingly relevant to next-generation BCIs for several reasons:

- **They support decision-making and reinforcement learning,** which are essential for adaptive BCIs and shared-autonomy interfaces.
- **They modulate emotional and physiological states,** enabling affect-aware BCIs and mental health interventions.
- **They form gating and control circuits for motor initiation,** which are critical for decoding intention or restoring movement in neurological disorders.

Although accessing subcortical signals is more challenging due to their depth, advances in deep-brain stimulation (DBS), high-resolution imaging, and bioelectronic implants are making these networks increasingly accessible for BCI applications.

### 2.1.3 Cortico–Subcortical Integration for BCI Systems

BCIs traditionally focus on cortical surface activity, but real-world cognition emerges from the interplay between cortical and subcortical circuits. Motor intention, emotion, memory, attention, and decision-making all depend on tightly coupled cortico–subcortical pathways. Nowadays, more BCI technology evolves toward decoding complex cognitive states and supporting adaptive closed-loop interactions, which makes it essential to incorporating deep regions of the brain. Thus, understanding brain organization from the layered structure of the cortex to the regulatory functions of subcortical nuclei can provide the foundation for interpreting neural signals and designing effective, reliable BCI systems.

## 2.2 The Brain in BCI: Structures and Signal Sources

### 2.2.1 The Cerebral Cortex and Its Role in BCIs

The cerebral cortex is the brain's highly folded outermost layer and provide many of the neural signals which is most relevant for BCI systems. As introduced earlier, it supports complex perceptual, cognitive, and motor processes that can be measured and decoded using invasive or noninvasive methods. The cortex is broadly divided into four major lobes—frontal, parietal, temporal, and occipital, as shown in Figure 2.3a. While referring to different parts of the human brain as per anatomical planes, specific terminology is utilized, shown in Figure 2.3b. Each of these

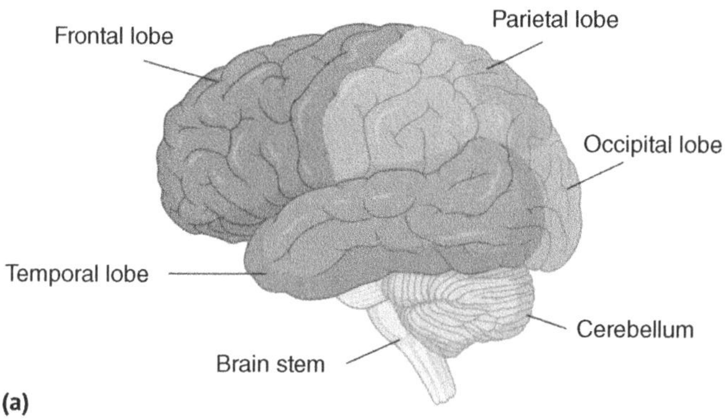


(a)

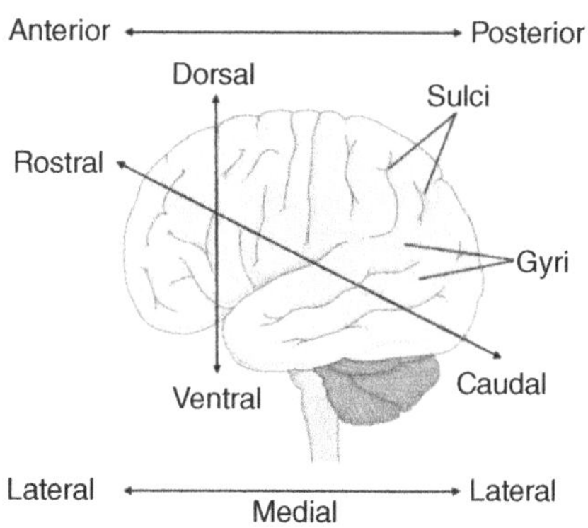


(b)

**Figure 2.3** Human brain lobes and their anatomical planes: (a) human brain lobes divided into frontal, parietal, occipital, and temporal lobe; (b) anatomical planes for human brain with "anterior" as in front of and toward the face and "posterior" as behind and toward the back; "medial" is toward the middle and "lateral" is toward the edge; "dorsal" as in top of the brain and "ventral" is toward the bottom of the brain; "rostral" is toward the front of the brain and "caudal" is toward the back of the brain.

regions are contributing distinct functional specializations (Figure 2.4). In addition to these primary layers, several specialized cortical regions also play important roles in emotion, conflict monitoring, and cognitive control. All of these cortical areas form the major source of neural activity known in BCI applications. Let us look at different brain regions and their corresponding roles for BCI.

#### 2.2.1.1 Frontal Lobe

The frontal lobe occupies the anterior portion of the cerebral cortex, which extends from the forehead region to the central sulcus. It is also the largest cortical region and is responsible for executive function, motor control, working memory, and decision-making. Many active BCI paradigms including those based on MI, intentional control, and cognitive workload estimation derive their signals from activity within this lobe. Key subregions of the frontal lobe include:

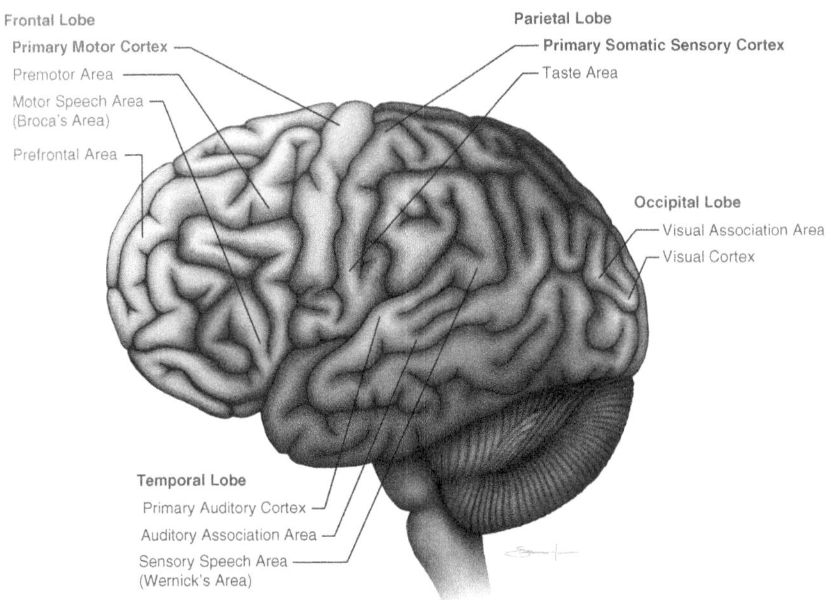


**Figure 2.4** Lateral view of the cerebral cortex showing major lobes and functional areas (motor, sensory, visual, auditory, language-related regions) based on Nicholas Margarot blog.

- **Primary Motor Cortex (M1):** M1 is located in the precentral gyrus immediately anterior to the central sulcus. It is the key cortical region responsible for initiating and controlling voluntary movements. It contains a somatotopic representation of the body, meaning different parts of the cortex correspond to specific muscle groups. M1 generates robust, high-frequency neural activity related to movement execution and imagined movement, making it one of the most widely used regions in motor action related BCIs. Both invasive systems such as intracortical microelectrode arrays and noninvasive approaches such as sensorimotor rhythms in EEG rely heavily on M1 activity to decode hand trajectories, grasp forces, or limb kinematics for prosthetic control and neurorehabilitation.
- **Premotor Cortex and Supplementary Motor Area (SMA):** Premotor cortex is located anterior to M1 on the lateral surface of the frontal lobe and SMA, found medially along the superior frontal gyrus. The premotor cortex is responsible for planning, preparing, and sequencing movements. These regions become active before movement onset, reflecting intention, action selection, and MI processes. Because their activity precedes and predicts movement, they are highly valuable for intent-driven BCIs, early movement detection, and systems requiring predictive control such as exoskeletons or robotic limbs. The SMA also contributes to internally generated actions and bimanual coordination, making it relevant for BCIs designed for stroke rehabilitation and motor recovery.
- **Prefrontal Cortex (PFC):** Occupying the anterior portion of the frontal lobe, the PFC integrates information from sensory, limbic, and motor systems to support executive functions, cognitive control, reasoning, and social behavior. It plays a major role in planning, decision-making, maintaining task goals, and regulating emotional responses. Because PFC activity reflects high-level cognitive states such as attention, workload, uncertainty, and intention, it is increasingly targeted in cognitive and affective BCIs. The PFC encompasses several important subdivisions, including the dorsolateral prefrontal cortex (DLPFC), ventromedial prefrontal cortex (vmPFC), orbitofrontal cortex (OFC), and anterior cingulate cortex (ACC). Each of these subdivisions contributes to working memory, impulse control, prediction, and performance monitoring. Major subdivisions related to BCIs are:
  - Dorsolateral Prefrontal Cortex (DLPFC): DLPFC is located on the lateral surface of the frontal lobe. It is known as a hub for executive control and high-level cognition. It supports working memory, planning, cognitive flexibility, and the maintenance of task goals. Its role in sustaining attention, managing complex sequences, and exerting top-down control makes it an important region for BCIs that track cognitive workload, monitor attentional engagement, or decode decision-related neural activity. The DLPFC

is also frequently targeted in passive BCIs that estimate mental effort or fatigue in real-world environments.

- Ventromedial Prefrontal Cortex (vmPFC): Situated along the medial and orbital surfaces of the frontal lobe, the vmPFC integrates emotional, motivational, and cognitive signals to guide value-based decision-making. It is responsible for reward processing, emotional regulation, preference formation, evaluating risk and uncertainty. Because vmPFC activity reflects internal affective and motivational states, it is increasingly relevant for affective BCIs, adaptive user interfaces, and systems that personalize responses based on user engagement, stress, or emotional context.
- Orbitofrontal Cortex (OFC): OFC is positioned on the ventral surface of the frontal lobe, above the eye orbits. It is an important part of the brain evaluating outcomes, adjusting behavior in a changing environment, and also integrating sensory and emotional cues. It is involved in impulse control, social behavior, and learning from reward and punishment. These functions make the OFC relevant for BCIs designed for adaptive reinforcement learning and neuropsychiatric intervention, where tracking evaluative or reward-based neural signals enhances prediction of user intent or internal state.

#### 2.2.1.2 Parietal Lobe

The parietal lobe lies posterior to the central sulcus and superior to the occipital lobe, forming the upper rear portion of the cerebral cortex. It plays a central role in integrating multisensory information, constructing spatial representations, guiding attention, and maintaining body awareness. These functions are essential for both reactive BCIs, which rely on stimulus-driven neural responses, and intent-based BCIs that decode voluntary motor goals or attentional states. The parietal lobe acts as a major hub for translating perception into action which is essential for naturalistic motor control and shared autonomy systems. Key regions within the parietal lobe include with respect to BCI:

##### *2.2.1.2.1 Primary Somatosensory Cortex (S1)*

S1 is located in the postcentral gyrus, posterior to the central sulcus. It contains a somatotopic map of the body and processes tactile, proprioceptive, and kinesthetic input. It also provides essential sensory feedback signals for BCIs related to prosthetic limbs, such as haptic feedback. Closed-loop BCIs can utilize this region to decode and stimulate the sense of touch, improve motor precision, and enhance artificial limb embodiments. Additionally, S1 is useful for BCIs for monitoring posture, limb position, and somatosensory attention.

#### 2.2.1.2.2 Posterior Parietal Cortex (PPC)

Situated in the superior and inferior parietal lobules behind S1, the PPC integrates visual, auditory, and somatosensory information to create high-level representations of spatial goals, target locations, and planned actions. It serves as a hub for sensorimotor transformation, converting sensory input into abstract motor intentions before motor commands are formed. Importantly, PPC activity can reveal user intent even without overt movement or strong MI signals, making it a powerful target for intuitive, goal-based BCIs. While the SMA also encodes movement intention and internally generated action plans, its activity is typically closer to motor execution and reflects sequencing or initiation of specific movements. In contrast, the PPC represents more abstract, high-level goals such as the desired direction or target before these are translated into motor programs, making it especially valuable for BCIs focused on goal decoding, shared autonomy, or predictive control.

### 2.2.1.3 Occipital Lobe

The occipital lobe is the posterior portion of the cerebral cortex, behind the parietal and temporal lobes. It is responsible for visual processing and interpreting information such as color, orientation, motion, and depth. Because visual perception generates strong and highly structured neural responses, the occipital lobe plays a central role in visual stimulus-based BCIs, including systems that rely on event-related potentials (ERPs), for example, P300 and steady-state visual evoked potentials (SSVEP). These paradigms exploit the robustness and reliability of visually evoked responses, making occipital regions an ideal target for high-speed, low-effort BCI communication and control. Key functional areas within the occipital lobe include:

#### 2.2.1.3.1 Primary Visual Cortex (V1)

Located along the calcarine sulcus on the medial surface of the occipital lobe, V1 is the first cortical region to receive visual input from the retina via the thalamus. It processes fundamental visual features such as orientation, spatial frequency, contrast, and direction of motion. V1 generates strong evoked potentials in response to flickering or patterned stimuli, forming the basis of many SSVEP-based BCIs. Because V1 exhibits precise retinotopic organization, BCIs can harness spatially distinct responses to multiple visual targets for multi-choice interfaces.

#### 2.2.1.3.2 Extrastriate Visual Areas (V2, V3, V4, etc.)

Surrounding V1, the extrastriate cortex comprises a hierarchy of visual areas that analyze increasingly complex aspects of visual scenes. Visual regions V2 and V3 are known to support contour integration, depth perception, and motion tracking. V4 is responsible for color processing, object features, and attention-related enhancements. These regions modulate visual evoked responses and play an important role in attentional selection, making them valuable for BCIs that rely on covert attention shifts, visually guided decision-making, or enhanced decoding of multifeature stimuli. Activity in extrastriate areas can improve classification accuracy in hybrid BCIs that combine SSVEP, P300, or eye-gaze information.

#### 2.2.1.4 Temporal Lobe

The temporal lobe is located on the lateral sides of the cerebral cortex, below the frontal and parietal lobes and adjacent to the ear. It is an important part of the brain in auditory perception, language comprehension, semantic processing, memory formation, and aspects of emotion regulation. Because auditory and linguistic stimuli evoke reliable neural signatures, the temporal lobe is highly relevant for auditory-based BCIs, speech or language decoding systems. Its regions also contribute to memory and emotion, enabling BCIs that monitor cognitive state, track learning, or interact with internal mental content. Key areas within the temporal lobe include:

##### *2.2.1.4.1 Primary Auditory Cortex (A1)*

A1 is located in the superior temporal gyrus and receives the first cortical projections from the auditory thalamus. It processes fundamental acoustic features such as pitch, rhythm, amplitude, and temporal modulation. It also generates auditory ERPs, popular with auditory oddball tasks, spatial hearing, and sonification-related paradigms, especially for users with limited visual inputs. It also supports hybrid BCIs, combining auditory cues with attention monitoring or speech imagery signals.

##### *2.2.1.4.2 Wernicke's Area*

Typically situated in the posterior portion of the left superior temporal gyrus, Wernicke's area is essential for language comprehension, semantic integration, and mapping auditory signals onto meaning. It plays a crucial role in auditory sentence processing and spoken word recognition. This region is increasingly explored in communication BCIs, especially those aimed at decoding imagined speech, auditory attention, or continuous speech representations. Its involvement in linguistic prediction and semantic context processing makes it valuable for BCIs aspiring to restore communication for individuals with severe motor or speech impairments.

##### *2.2.1.4.3 Medial Temporal Lobe (MTL)*

MTL is located on the inner surface of the temporal lobe and consists of the hippocampus, entorhinal cortex, and parahippocampal gyrus. These areas are fundamental for episodic memory formation, spatial navigation, and consolidation of long-term memories. Because MTL neurons exhibit well-characterized activity patterns including place cells, grid cells, and concept cells, this region is a promising target for memory-based BCIs, neural prosthetics for memory restoration, and cognitive monitoring systems. MTL activity can also support BCIs related to mental imagery and spatial navigation, therefore allowing interaction with deeper cognitive processes.

#### 2.2.1.5 Insular Cortex

The insula, or insular cortex, lies deep within the lateral sulcus, beneath the frontal, temporal, and parietal lobes. It serves as a multimodal integration hub that brings together sensory, visceral, emotional, and cognitive information. Functionally, the insula plays a central role in interoception, which is the perception of internal bodily states, emotion processing, risk evaluation, social affect, and the subjective feeling of bodily ownership. These capabilities make it highly relevant to BCIs that aim to measure or modulate internal emotional states, stress levels, or physiological arousal. The anterior insula contributes to awareness of salience and affect, supporting BCIs designed for emotion tracking, adaptive workload management, or mental-state recognition in real-world environments. The posterior insula, which processes somatosensory and visceral input, can be leveraged in BCIs focused on autonomic monitoring or pain detection. As interest grows in affective BCIs and closed-loop neuroadaptive systems, the insula is becoming a key target for decoding internal states that influence decision-making, performance, and user engagement.

#### 2.2.1.6 Cingulate Cortex

The cingulate cortex is located on the medial surface of the cerebral hemispheres, covering the corpus callosum. This is an important part of the limbic system, therefore involved with emotion, motivation, attention control, and cognitive regulation. Its anatomical and functional subdivisions play distinct roles in BCI applications:

##### *2.2.1.6.1 Anterior Cingulate Cortex (ACC)*

Located in the frontal portion of the cingulate gyrus, the ACC is central to performance monitoring, conflict detection, decision-making under uncertainty, and emotional regulation. It generates characteristic error-related potentials (ErrPs) in EEG signals when a user perceives a mistake or mismatch, a signal widely leveraged in adaptive BCIs for automatic error correction, shared autonomy, and feedback optimization. ACC activity also reflects effort allocation, sustained attention, and motivational drive, enabling BCIs that monitor cognitive fatigue, engagement, or stress during long-duration tasks.

#### *2.2.1.6.2 Posterior Cingulate Cortex (PCC)*

Situated in the posterior part of the cingulate gyrus, the PCC is a core node of the default mode network (DMN) and is strongly associated with internally directed thought, mind-wandering, autobiographical memory, and self-referential processing. The PCC plays an important role in regulating transitions between internal and external attention, making it relevant for passive BCIs aimed at detecting lapses in attention, monitoring mental workload, or assessing vigilance levels. PCC activities are known to be correlated with cognitive states such as mental fatigue, drowsiness, and mind-wondering, etc. Therefore, they can support the development of BCIs where sustained attention or cognitive engagement is required.

One of the major advantages of targeting cortical regions is their accessibility closer to the scalp. Noninvasive neuroimaging techniques such as EEG, MEG, and fNIRS rely on scalp-based recording that can access cortical activities, therefore opening the possibility to develop portable and user-friendly BCIs without needing surgical intervention. For applications demanding higher spatial and temporal resolution, invasive methods like ECoG or intracortical microelectrode arrays can provide detailed access to cortical dynamics at the level of neuronal populations or even single neurons. Due to its critical role in both cognitive processing and signal accessibility, the cerebral cortex remains the primary neural substrate for most current BCI applications spanning clinical tools and consumer technologies. Ongoing research into cortical oscillations, functional connectivity, and neuroplasticity continues to improve the precision, adaptability, and robustness of BCI systems, with significant impact in areas such as neurorehabilitation, assistive communication, cognitive enhancement, and mental health monitoring.

## 2.2.2 Beyond the Cortex: Subcortical and Distributed Networks

BCIs majorly target the cerebral cortex to access and intercept brain activities; however, several subcortical structures and distributed brain networks also play critical roles in cognitive functions. These deeper structures, as shown in Figure 2.5, are essential for processes such as decision-making, learning, emotion regulation, and motor coordination. These functions are increasingly relevant to next-generation BCI applications.

### 2.2.2.1 Basal Ganglia

The basal ganglia are a group of nuclei situated deep within the cerebral hemispheres, heavily involved in action selection, habit formation, and motor control. They interface extensively with cortical areas via the cortico-basal ganglia-thalamo-cortical loops, making them vital for both voluntary and automatic motor behaviors. BCIs targeting motor planning, error detection, or reinforcement-based

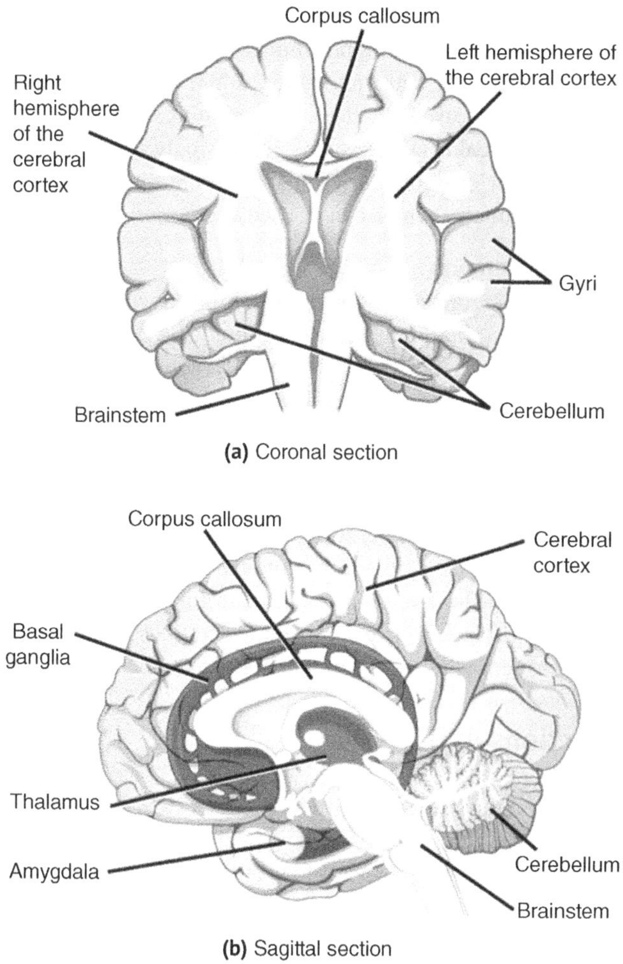


**Figure 2.5** These illustrations show the (a) coronal and (b) sagittal sections of the human brain.

learning increasingly consider the modulatory influence of basal ganglia activity, particularly in applications like prosthetic control and neurorehabilitation in BCIs.

#### 2.2.2.2 Thalamus

The thalamus acts as a central relay station, routing sensory information to appropriate cortical areas and regulating attentional gating. It supports oscillatory synchronization between cortical and subcortical regions and is implicated in consciousness, alertness, and working memory. Disruptions in thalamic function can significantly impact EEG rhythms, making it relevant for interpreting neural signatures in attention-modulated or consciousness-related BCIs.

#### 2.2.2.3 Limbic System

The limbic system, including the amygdala, hippocampus, and parts of the cingulate cortex, is central to emotional processing, motivation, and memory formation. Emotion-aware BCIs, such as those used in affective computing, mental health monitoring, or immersive virtual reality (VR) systems, increasingly rely on signals influenced by limbic activity. For example, amygdala-based emotional salience can modulate frontal alpha asymmetry, which can be used in emotion-based BCIs.

#### 2.2.2.4 Distributed Functional Networks

Modern cognitive neuroscience emphasizes that most mental functions emerge from distributed neural networks rather than isolated regions. The DMN, salience network, and frontoparietal control network dynamically coordinate activity across brain regions during rest, attention, or cognitive switching tasks. Understanding functional brain networks could be very useful for BCI development, where the aim is to assess internal mental states such as fatigue, engagement, and cognitive load. Additionally, incorporating the subcortical and distributed networks allows understanding of how different parts of the brain communicate in real-time, thereby facilitating the development of context-aware, adaptive, and perhaps emotionally intelligent BCIs. The progress in neuroimaging techniques along with machine learning (ML) may help to access brain activities in the deeper brain structure, therefore broadening the scope of BCI applications.

## 2.3 Cognitive Functions in BCI

BCIs aim to detect and respond to specific cognitive functions such as attention, motor control, memory, emotion, and decision-making. As we have seen in the previous section, BCIs aim to detect and respond to cognitive functions such as attention, motor control, emotion, decision-making, etc. These functions collectively constitute the equivalent of "WHAT" in a BCI system, which allows interpretable neural signals from cognitive processes. Each known cognitive function can be represented by a unique set of neural features which can be decoded from the recorded electrophysiological or hemodynamic recording techniques. As a result, BCI systems can extract information about mental state or intention or control and translate them into real-time commands or feedback to form the "HOW." While some cognitive functions are still being explored in terms of their neurophysiological correlates and practical decoding methods, several have been well-characterized and successfully implemented in real-world applications. Understanding these cognitive processes and how they map onto specific neural signals is essential for building BCIs that are not only functional but also adaptive, intuitive, and user-centered. In the following subsections, we explore key cognitive domains that have proven particularly relevant for BCI development, along with the associated brain regions, neural markers, and application areas.

### 2.3.1 Attention Function

The attention system enables individuals to prioritize certain stimuli over others, supporting goal-directed behavior by filtering irrelevant information. Attention is reflected in a unique neural signature that can be decoded to reflect whether a user is consciously or unconsciously attending to a stimulus. One of the most commonly known neural signatures for attention is P300, which is an ERP in EEG signals that occurs at 300 ms post significant or unique stimulus presentation. P300 is known to be found in oddball paradigms where users identify rare or target items among frequent distractors. An example could be seeing an elephant, which elicits P300 among a set of pictures of sea animals. P300-based BCIs are widely implemented in speller systems, allowing users to make selections without physical movement.

Another robust attention marker is the SSVEP, which is generated when a person focuses on a flickering visual stimulus; however, similar effect can be achieved by auditory and tactile flickering as well. Sometimes also known as steady-state evoked potential (SSxEP) where x could be visual, auditory, or tactile stimuli. When SSxEP presented to user, the brain's response in occipital lobe aligns with the flicker frequency, enabling reliable decoding for high-speed, real-time applications.

Alpha-band desynchronization (8–12 Hz), especially over parietal and occipital areas, is also associated with attentional engagement. These patterns are useful in systems that monitor sustained attention or fatigue, including driver alertness monitors, e-learning tools, and human–robot interfaces.

In recent years, researchers also explore hybrid BCIs that combine ERP, spectral, and hemodynamic signals (e.g., fNIRS or fMRI) to improve robustness and minimize calibration requirements.

### 2.3.2 Motor Function

Motor function is a foundational area in BCI research due to its well-understood neural basis and clinical relevance. It involves neural activity related to the planning, execution, or imagination of movement, typically originating from the primary motor cortex (M1), supplementary motor area (SMA), and premotor cortex. Motor BCIs primarily use two strategies:

- **Motor execution**: In these BCI systems, neural activity is measured during actual physical movement, typically using EEG or ECoG. While effective, this approach is less suitable for users with severe motor impairments.
- **Motor imagery (MI)**: MI occurs when a user imagines a movement of a specific body part such as legs, hands, or fingers. Such an imagined movement generally results in suppression of mu (8–13 Hz) and beta (13–30 Hz)

rhythms over sensorimotor areas with unique patterns for different imagined movements.

MI BCIs are widely used in stroke rehabilitation, stimulating neuroplasticity to aid recovery. They are also employed in prosthetic control and robotic interface systems. Emerging systems integrate MI with real-time multimodal feedback (visual, tactile, proprioceptive) to form closed-loop BCIs, enhancing learning and performance.

### 2.3.3 Decision-making Function

Decision-making encompasses the cognitive processes involved in selecting actions or responses based on context, prior experience, goals, and emotional input. It involves a distributed network that includes the PFC, ACC, and basal ganglia. BCIs interpret decision-making processes through the following neuro markers:

- **Error-related potentials (ErrPs)**: Negative ERP components that occur approximately 200 ms, also known as N200 when a user perceives an error, either self-generated or produced by the system. These signals are valuable in error correction mechanisms, allowing the BCI to adapt based on detected user dissatisfaction.
- **Readiness potentials (Bereitschaftspotential)**: Readiness potentials are slow cortical potentials that precede voluntary movement, also known as Bereitschaftspotential in German where it was found. These potentials can be used to predict a user's intent and are commonly used in combination with MI for BCI-based control systems.
- **Theta and beta oscillations**: Modulations in theta and beta frequency bands are associated with task difficulty, decision uncertainty, and cognitive control processes.

These functions have wide variety of applications including adaptive gaming, neuroadaptive decision aids, and shared control systems such as semi-autonomous vehicles and robotic arms where user intention supplements autonomous behavior. These are particularly valuable when traditional input methods are unreliable or unavailable.

### 2.3.4 Emotion Function

Emotions significantly influence cognitive processes including attention, learning, and decision-making. Emotion processing involves a distributed network including the amygdala, insula, ACC, and vmPFC. Emotion-aware BCIs rely on physiological and neural indicators such as:

- **Frontal alpha asymmetry**: Left-dominant activity is linked to positive emotion, while right-dominant is linked to negative affect.
- **EEG spectral features**: Increased theta and beta activity during stress, anxiety, or cognitive engagement.
- **Multimodal integration**: Combining EEG with heart rate variability (HRV), galvanic skin response (GSR), and facial electromyogram (EMG) improves classification.

These neural indicators are popularly used in BCIs for affective computing and biofeedback therapy.

### 2.3.5 Executive Function

It is a group of high-level cognitive processes that are essential for goal-directed behavior. They enable individuals to set objectives, plan and organize actions, make decisions, regulate impulses, adapt to changing circumstances, and monitor ongoing performance. These functions are critical for maintaining focus, managing multiple tasks, inhibiting inappropriate responses, and flexibly shifting between mental states or strategies. Some executive functions have neural correlates, which can be used in BCIs:

- **Working memory**: Temporarily holding and manipulating information.
- **Inhibitory control**: Suppressing irrelevant or inappropriate responses.
- **Cognitive flexibility**: Shifting between tasks or mental frameworks.

Neuroanatomically, these executive functions are primarily mediated by the PFC, particularly the dorsolateral, ventrolateral, and anterior cingulate regions, which interact with subcortical structures to support adaptive behavior. To detect these executive functions, BCIs utilize the following correlates:

- **Midfrontal theta activity**: It reflects the change in cognitive control, associated with coordination of goal-directed behaviors in task involving action monitoring, error detection, prediction, and updating an ongoing strategy.
- **Components of ERPs**: Related to attention such as P300 and conflict monitoring such as N200. These ERP components are associated with unexpected or task-relevant events, which are also related to attention and cognitive control, similar to mid-frontal theta activity but in the time domain.
- **Alpha suppression**: Indicates mental effort and engagement. Reduced alpha power is often observed when individuals direct attention, process complex information, or sustain heightened readiness for action.

Executive function-based BCIs are used in neurofeedback training for attention-deficit/hyperactivity disorder (ADHD), cognitive workload monitoring in safety-critical domains, and resilience training in high-stress environments. With improvements in decoding and wearable technologies, these applications are becoming more scalable and user-centric.

## 2.4 Neural Correlates: The "HOW" of Cognitive Decoding

Neural correlates are the measurable signals representing cognitive activity using invasive or noninvasive sensing. Neural basis and correlates of cognitive functions form the "**how**" to use the brain signals to create BCIs. Let's look at the summary Table 2.1.

**Table 2.1** Cognitive functions, their neural correlates, and representative BCI applications.

| Cognitive function | Neural correlates | BCI applications |
|---|---|---|
| Attention | P300, SSVEP, Alpha suppression | Spellers, attention-aware interfaces, vigilance monitoring |
| MI | Mu/Beta rhythm suppression | Robotic control, neurorehabilitation, prosthetic devices |
| Working memory | Theta power, Alpha modulation, ERP | Adaptive learning, workload monitoring, performance prediction |
| Emotion | Frontal alpha asymmetry, beta/theta activity | Affective BCIs, mood tracking, mental health monitoring |
| Error detection | Error-related negativity (ERN), P300 | Adaptive correction, error-aware feedback systems |
| Decision-making | Slow cortical potentials, theta/beta oscillations | Preference prediction, shared control, neuroadaptive systems |
| Sensory processing | SSVEP, P300, ERP | Stimulus detection, high-speed spellers, attention decoding |
| Executive functions | Midfrontal theta, PFC activity, P300 | Cognitive workload estimation, ADHD training, executive monitoring |
| Language processing | N400, P600, left-hemisphere ERPs | Communication BCIs, speech restoration, semantic conflict detection |

| Cognitive function | Neural correlates | BCI applications |
|---|---|---|
| Learning | Feedback-related negativity (FRN), dopamine-mediated rhythms | Closed-loop BCIs, reinforcement learning interfaces, neurofeedback |
| Social cognition | Medial PFC activity, ERP markers of perspective-taking | Adaptive interfaces, empathy-based systems, human-robot collaboration |
| Fatigue and drowsiness | Alpha/theta ratio, vigilance ERPs | Driver alertness, sustained attention systems, safety-critical monitoring |

## 2.5 Summary

In this chapter, we explored how the cerebral cortex, especially motor, sensory, and prefrontal regions, serves as a primary source of neural signals used in BCI systems. Furthermore, we highlighted the importance of subcortical structures and distributed brain networks in supporting complex functions such as emotion, learning, and decision-making, which are now becoming integral to advanced BCI applications. By identifying neural correlates of specific cognitive functions such as attention, MI, working memory, and emotion, BCIs can translate them into actionable outputs. These functions define the "what" of BCI systems, while the neural correlates and signal acquisition methods define the "how."

A deep understanding of these relationships enables the development of more adaptive, intuitive, and personalized BCI systems. As the field advances, the integration of cognitive neuroscience, neurotechnology, and ML will continue to expand the boundaries of what BCIs can achieve across healthcare, communication, education, and human–machine interaction.

# 3

# Acquisition and Stimulation Technology

Our understanding of the brain was historically shaped by behavioral observations, psychological studies, and analyses based on responses to external stimuli. Before the advent of brain sensing technologies, most insights into brain function came from clinical observation or trial-and-error approaches, which often involved individuals with brain injuries. For instance, damage to the temporal lobe can impair speech, while injury to the visual cortex may result in vision loss. These early, often accidental findings laid the groundwork for associating specific brain regions with distinct cognitive and motor functions, helping to map the brain's architecture through indirect evidence.

Modern advances in neuroscience and brain–computer interfaces (BCIs) have been driving the development of neurotechnologies, particularly acquisition and stimulation technologies. Acquisition technologies capture and measure neural activity, translating brain signals into data that BCI systems can interpret. They form the input side of the interface, enabling machines to "listen" to the brain in real time. Stimulation technologies, in contrast, provide the output channel by delivering targeted signals to the brain or nervous system to influence activity, evoke specific responses, or offer feedback, enabling so-called "writing" to the brain. Together, these technologies enable dynamic, two-way interaction between the brain and external systems, transforming BCIs from passive monitoring tools into adaptive, functional platforms with applications in communication, control, rehabilitation, and therapy. This chapter delves into these technologies in detail.

## 3.1 Invasive and Noninvasive Acquisition Technologies in BCI

The introduction of brain sensing mechanisms marked a major turning point in cognitive neuroscience. The development of technologies capable of directly capturing brain activity in both invasive and noninvasive enabled researchers to study the brain in real time. Unlike earlier methods, these tools support continuous and dynamic observation of neural processes under both controlled and natural conditions. These acquisition technologies form the foundation of modern BCI systems by translating neural signals into actionable data for communication, control, and rehabilitation. Broadly, they can be classified into noninvasive and invasive approaches, each offering distinct advantages and limitations. Noninvasive techniques emphasize safety and ease of use, while invasive methods offer higher signal fidelity and spatial resolution. The following sections explore these brain signal acquisition techniques in detail.

### 3.1.1 Noninvasive Acquisition Technologies

Noninvasive brain signal acquisition techniques are widely used in BCI research due to their safety, portability, and ease of application. These methods do not require surgical intervention and are generally more acceptable for long-term or daily use. However, they often come with trade-offs, such as lower spatial resolution and increased susceptibility to noise. Figure 3.1 illustrates five widely available noninvasive technologies, with details provided below.

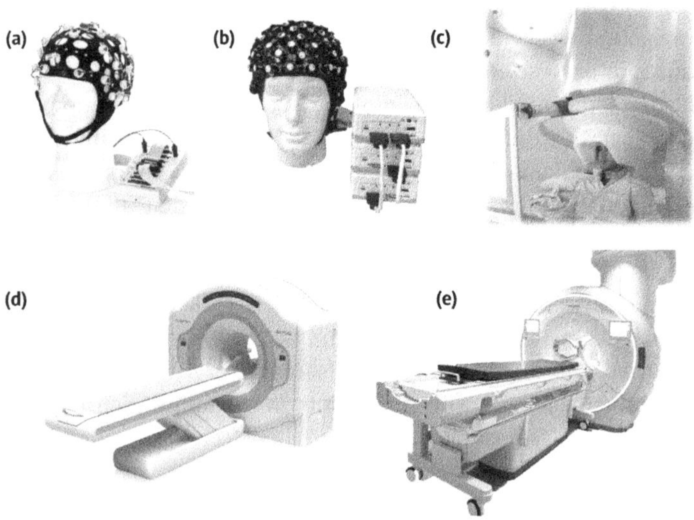


**Figure 3.1** Noninvasive acquisition devices: (a) Electroencephalography (EEG), (b) Functional Near-infrared Spectroscopy (fNIRS), (c) Magnetoencephalography (MEG), *Source*: https://commons.wikimedia.org/wiki/File:NIMH_MEG.jpg/last accessed Dec. 22, 2025/Public domain (d) Positron Emission Tomography (PET), *Source*: Spacecoastcreative/Wikimedia Common/https://commons.wikimedia.org/wiki/File:Positron_emission_tomography.png/last accessed Dec. 22, 2025/CC-0, and (e) Functional Magnetic Resonance Imaging (fMRI).

#### 3.1.1.1 Electroencephalography

Electroencephalography (EEG) measures the brain's electrical activity through electrodes placed on the scalp. The electrical signals originate from post-synaptic potentials generated by large groups of pyramidal neurons in the cortex. These potentials create voltage fluctuations that can be detected at the scalp surface. EEG systems typically use conductive gel or dry electrode interfaces to ensure proper signal conduction. The signals are recorded across multiple channels, representing different regions of the brain, and are then filtered and processed to extract relevant features such as frequency bands or event-related potentials.

EEG is one of the most established and widely used techniques in BCI research due to its excellent temporal resolution, low cost, and ease of deployment. It is particularly well suited for real-time applications such as MI-based control, attention monitoring, and affective state detection. Despite its widespread use, EEG suffers from low spatial resolution because the signals must pass through the skull and scalp, leading to spatial smearing. Additionally, it is prone to artifacts caused by muscle movements, eye blinks, and external electrical interference.

#### 3.1.1.2 Functional Near-infrared Spectroscopy

Functional near-infrared spectroscopy (fNIRS) uses near-infrared light to measure changes in blood oxygenation levels within the cortex. Light in the near-infrared range (approximately 700–900 nanometers) can penetrate the skull and interact with oxygenated and deoxygenated hemoglobin in the blood. Light emitters and detectors are placed on the scalp, and the system calculates relative concentrations of hemoglobin by analyzing the absorption and scattering of the light as it travels through the brain tissue.

This technique indirectly reflects neural activity based on the principle of neurovascular coupling, where increased neuronal activity leads to localized increases in blood flow and oxygen delivery. While fNIRS offers better spatial localization than EEG and is less sensitive to electrical noise, its temporal resolution is limited due to the slow nature of hemodynamic responses. Nonetheless, fNIRS is gaining popularity in BCI applications related to cognitive workload assessment, mental state monitoring, and brain-based communication, particularly in settings where noninvasiveness and mobility are critical.

#### 3.1.1.3 Magnetoencephalography

Magnetoencephalography (MEG) measures the magnetic fields generated by electrical currents associated with neuronal activity, primarily from synchronous firing of pyramidal neurons in the cortex. These magnetic fields are extremely weak on the order of femtoteslas and are detected using highly sensitive devices known as superconducting quantum interference devices (SQUIDs) or optically pumped magnetometers (OPMs). Unlike EEG, magnetic fields are not distorted by the skull and scalp, allowing MEG to provide better spatial accuracy while retaining excellent temporal resolution. MEG signals are recorded from multiple channels in a shielded room to eliminate background magnetic noise. The system reconstructs the sources of brain activity using advanced signal processing and source localization algorithms.

Despite its advantages, MEG remains limited to research and specialized clinical environments due to its high cost, lack of portability, and complex operational requirements. It is used to investigate brain dynamics, functional connectivity, and cortical mapping in experimental BCI studies. However, there are known attempts to reduce the size of MEG by researchers around the world, which may open up significant number of possibilities in BCIs.

#### 3.1.1.4 Functional Magnetic Resonance Imaging

Functional magnetic resonance imaging (fMRI) detects changes in brain activity by measuring blood oxygen level-dependent (BOLD) signals. Neural activation leads to localized increases in oxygenated blood flow, and fMRI captures these changes using a strong magnetic field and radiofrequency pulses. The difference in magnetic properties between oxygenated and deoxygenated hemoglobin results in varying signal intensities, which can be interpreted as indirect markers of neural activity. The primary strength of fMRI lies in its high spatial resolution, allowing detailed mapping of brain regions involved in specific tasks. fMRI data is acquired in volumes over time, creating a time series that reveals activation patterns during cognitive or sensory processing. However, its temporal resolution is poor due to the sluggish nature of hemodynamic responses, and the technique requires subjects to remain motionless inside a large and noisy scanner.

Due to its operational complexity and limited real-time capability, fMRI is mainly used for experimental research, brain mapping, and validation of other BCI modalities rather than direct BCI control. fMRI is also actively used to establish neural-basis of different cognitive functions, which is useful for develop BCIs.

#### 3.1.1.5 Positron Emission Tomography

Positron emission tomography (PET) is another noninvasive neuroimaging technique that measures metabolic activity in the brain using radiotracers, most commonly fluorodeoxyglucose (FDG). After a small amount of the tracer is injected into the bloodstream, it emits positrons that interact with electrons in nearby tissue, producing gamma rays that are detected by the scanner. The resulting images show glucose consumption or other metabolic processes, providing insight into regional brain activity. However, unlike EEG and MEG, which directly measure electrophysiological signals, PET reflects slower metabolic changes similar to fMRI and therefore has poor temporal resolution. However, it offers valuable information about neurochemical processes, neurotransmitter dynamics, and long-term metabolic patterns that are not accessible through other modalities. PET is frequently used in research involving cognitive function, neurodegenerative diseases, and functional brain mapping.

Due to these limitations, PET is not typically used for real-time control in BCI due to its low temporal resolution, cost, and the requirement for radioactive tracers. However, it plays an important role in validating neural mechanisms, identifying functional networks, and providing complementary physiological information that can guide the design and interpretation of BCI systems.

### 3.1.2 Invasive Acquisition Technologies

Invasive acquisition methods involve surgically implanting electrodes into or on the surface of the brain to capture neural signals with high spatial and temporal resolution. These methods bypass the filtering effects of the skull and scalp, allowing for more precise recordings. However, they are associated with higher risks, including infection, tissue damage, and long-term maintenance challenges. Most commonly available invasive acquisition technologies are shown in Figure 3.2.

#### 3.1.2.1 Intracortical Electrodes (Utah Array)

The Utah Array is a high-density grid composed of rigid microelectrodes that penetrate the cortical surface. Each electrode records extracellular potentials from individual neurons or small neural populations. These signals include action potentials and local field potentials, which are critical for decoding fine motor intentions or sensory feedback. This method enables the capture of highly detailed, high-frequency neural signals that are suitable for controlling robotic limbs, computer cursors, or other assistive devices in real time. The array is implanted through open-brain surgery and typically interfaces with external processing systems through percutaneous connectors or wirelessly. Although it offers state-of-the-art performance in signal quality, concerns remain regarding its long-term biocompatibility, electrode degradation, and patient safety.

#### 3.1.2.2 Electrocorticography

Electrocorticography (ECoG) involves placing a grid or strip of electrodes directly on the cortical surface, typically beneath the dura mater (subdural) or above it (epidural). It captures electrical potentials generated by groups of neurons, providing a signal quality that is superior to EEG and more stable over time than intracortical electrodes. The surgical procedure for ECoG is less invasive than penetrating implants, and the technique strikes a balance between signal resolution and surgical risk. ECoG allows for both spontaneous and evoked brain activity recording, and it is frequently used in clinical applications such as epilepsy localization. In BCIs, ECoG has been successfully applied in communication systems and motor prosthetics, especially where high performance is required with moderate invasiveness.

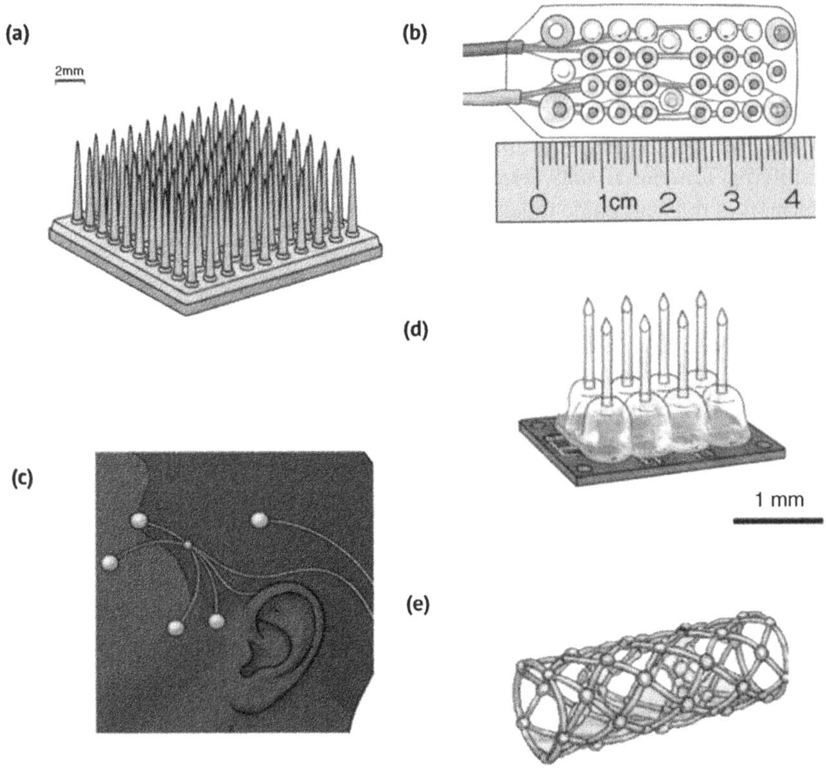


**Figure 3.2 Invasive acquisition devices illustration** (a) Utah Array, (b) electrocorticography (ECoG) grid, (c) stereo-electroencephalography (sEEG) depth electrodes, (d) Optogenetic probes, and (e) Stentrode.

### 3.1.2.3 Deep Brain Electrodes (Stereo-EEG)

Stereo-EEG or sEEG involves the stereotactic implantation of thin electrodes into deep brain structures to monitor electrical activity from regions such as the thalamus, amygdala, or hippocampus. These electrodes record local field potentials and are primarily used for epilepsy monitoring and presurgical planning.

In BCI applications, stereo-EEG allows researchers to explore cognitive and affective processes occurring in subcortical areas that are inaccessible to surface techniques. Although it provides rich neural data, its clinical use is limited due to its highly invasive nature and associated surgical risks. It is mainly applied in research settings and in patient populations undergoing neurosurgical evaluation.

#### 3.1.2.4 Optogenetic Probes

Optogenetics is a hybrid technique that combines genetic engineering with optical stimulation. Neurons are modified to express light sensitive ion channels, typically through viral vectors. Once targeted neurons express these proteins, their activity can be precisely controlled using specific wavelengths of light delivered via implanted optical fibers. In addition to stimulation, optogenetics can also be used for recording purposes when combined with genetically encoded indicators of neural activity. This approach allows for cellular-level precision in activating or silencing neural populations. While optogenetics has revolutionized neuroscience research in animal models, its application in human BCIs is still at an early experimental stage due to ethical and technical challenges related to gene delivery and long-term safety.

#### 3.1.2.5 Stentrode

The Stentrode is a novel, minimally invasive neural interface designed to be implanted through the vascular system, specifically targeting blood vessels near motor cortical regions. Delivered via a catheter, the device expands like a stent and anchors itself to the vessel wall, with embedded electrodes making contact with the endothelium.

Once in place, the Stentrode records electrocorticographic signals without the need for open-brain surgery. The device is connected to an external telemetry unit via a subcutaneous lead, enabling wireless transmission of brain signals. Early trials have demonstrated its feasibility for BCI control in individuals with severe paralysis, offering a promising alternative that combines safety with signal quality and long-term usability.

### 3.1.3 Comparison of Acquisition Techniques

Brain signal acquisition methods differ widely in how they balance spatial resolution, temporal resolution, portability, invasiveness, signal quality, and system complexity. These trade-offs strongly influence their suitability for different BCI applications. Figure 3.3 summarizes the relative positioning of common techniques across these dimensions with detailed below:

#### 3.1.3.1 Spatial Resolution

Spatial resolution determines how precisely a method can localize neural activity. Techniques such as intracortical electrodes and optogenetic probes offer the highest spatial precision, often resolving activity at the level of individual neurons. ECoG provides mesoscale spatial resolution by capturing population-level neural activity directly from the cortical surface. Among noninvasive methods, fMRI offers excellent spatial precision (millimeter scale), followed by MEG, which

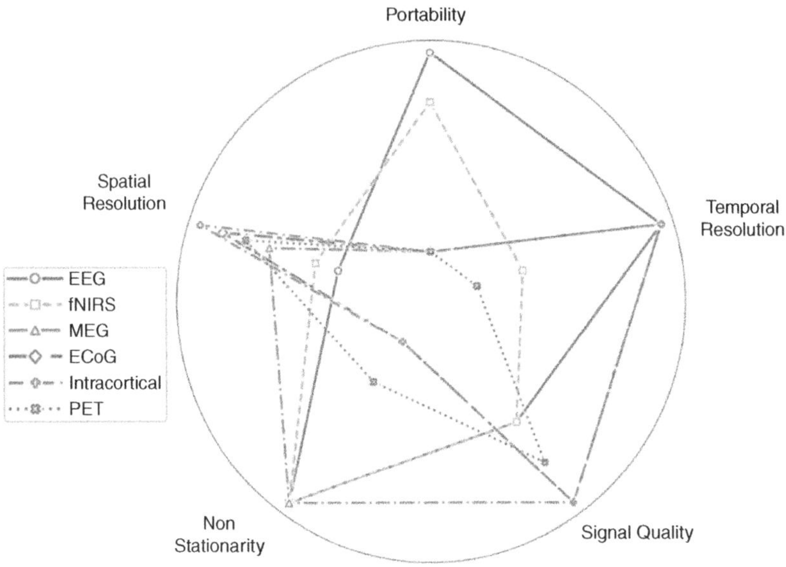


**Figure 3.3** Comparing brain imaging technologies based on their temporal, spatial resolution, portability, system complexity, noninvasiveness, and signal quality.

achieves good cortical localization due to minimal distortion of magnetic fields. EEG and fNIRS provide coarse spatial information, limited by volume conduction and diffusion of optical signals, respectively.

### 3.1.3.2 Temporal Resolution

Temporal resolution is critical for real-time BCIs and tracking fast neural dynamics. EEG, MEG, ECoG, and intracortical electrodes all provide millisecond-level resolution, making them well suited for continuous control of prosthetics, motor imagery BCIs, and rapid feedback systems. In contrast, hemodynamic techniques such as fMRI and fNIRS offer much slower temporal resolution (on the order of seconds) due to the nature of neurovascular coupling. These methods are better suited for cognitive state monitoring or communication systems where speed is less critical.

### 3.1.3.3 Portability and Practicality

Portability heavily influences real-world deployment. EEG and fNIRS are the most portable and user-friendly noninvasive modalities, allowing for mobile, wearable, and long-term monitoring systems. MEG and fMRI require large, stationary equipment housed in specialized facilities, significantly limiting their usability in daily-life BCIs. Recent developments in OPMs have demonstrated the potential for more compact and mobile MEG systems, but these remain largely experimental [55]. Among invasive methods, the Stentrode and newer wireless intracortical devices offer greater potential for long-term, home-based use compared to traditional tethered systems.

#### 3.1.3.4 Signal Quality and Robustness

Signal-to-noise ratio (SNR) and robustness to artifacts are major considerations in BCI performance. Intracortical electrodes yield the highest SNR, enabling fine-grained motor decoding. ECoG provides more reliable and stable recordings than scalp EEG while avoiding direct penetration of brain tissue. Noninvasive techniques such as EEG are more susceptible to environmental noise, movement artifacts, and physiological interference, whereas fNIRS is relatively robust but still affected by systemic factors such as skin blood flow.

#### 3.1.3.5 Invasiveness and Safety

Noninvasive techniques pose minimal risk and are suitable for widespread use, including healthy participants. Invasive technologies provide superior signal fidelity but require neurosurgery and carry risks such as infection, scarring, and long-term biocompatibility challenges. For this reason, highly invasive approaches such as intracortical arrays are typically limited to clinical populations with severe motor impairments.

### 3.1.4 Stimulation Technologies

In parallel with brain signal acquisition, stimulation technologies have emerged as an equally vital component of BCI development. While acquiring brain signals is what brings BCI systems to life enabling interaction with external devices and, on the other hand, stimulation technologies add a crucial interactive dimension. These technologies aim to deliver targeted signals to the brain or peripheral nervous system to influence, enhance, or modulate neural activity, making BCIs truly bidirectional systems. Although still relatively limited outside clinical settings, stimulation techniques have shown great promise in therapeutic interventions, motor function restoration, cognitive modulation, and adaptive feedback. By enabling BCIs to not only interpret but also meaningfully interact with brain activity, these technologies are transforming neuroscience from passive observation into active, two-way engagement. Together, acquisition and stimulation technologies are expanding our understanding of the brain and opening new pathways to restore, enhance, or even extend human capabilities. Let us now take a closer look at these acquisition technologies, also see Figure 3.4.

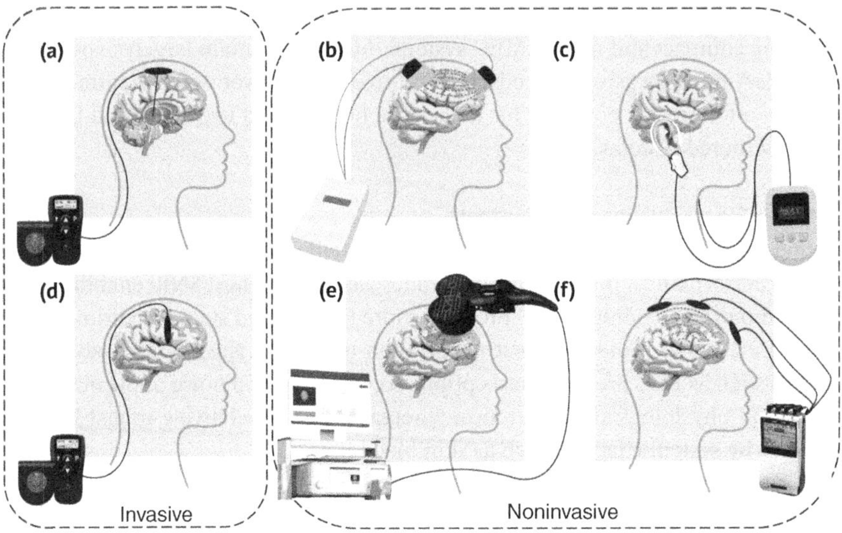


**Figure 3.4** Brain stimulation technologies based on: (a) deep brain stimulation (DBS); (b) Transcranial alternative/direct current stimulation (txCS); (c) Cranial electrotherapy stimulation; (d) Motor cortex stimulation; (e) Transcranial magnetic stimulation (TMS); (f) Reduced impedance noninvasive cortical electrostimulation. *Source*: [56]/Springer Nature/CC BY 4.0.

#### 3.1.4.1 Noninvasive Brain Stimulation

These techniques refer to a group of methods that influence brain activity through external devices applied to the scalp, without the need for surgical intervention. These methods aim to modulate cortical excitability and neural oscillations using magnetic or electrical fields and are commonly used for cognitive enhancement, neurorehabilitation, and research experiments.

##### *3.1.4.1.1 Transcranial Magnetic Stimulation*

Transcranial Magnetic Stimulation (TMS) uses magnetic fields to induce electrical currents in specific brain areas by placing a coil near the scalp. When a rapid current flows through the coil, it generates a magnetic field that passes through the skull and induces a secondary electric current in the underlying brain tissue. This current alters the excitability of neurons in the targeted region. TMS is used for both research and clinical treatments, including depression and motor recovery. It is noninvasive and can modulate cortical excitability, making it useful for neurorehabilitation and cognitive enhancement.

##### 3.1.4.1.2 Transcranial Direct Current Stimulation

Transcranial direct current stimulation (tDCS) applies a low constant electrical current through electrodes placed on the scalp. The current flows between an anode and a cathode, subtly altering the membrane potential of underlying neurons. This modulation can increase or decrease neuronal excitability depending on the polarity of the stimulation. tDCS is inexpensive, portable, and used to improve learning, attention, and mood. Although the exact mechanisms are still being studied, it holds promise for augmenting BCI performance and enhancing user engagement.

##### 3.1.4.1.3 Transcranial Alternating Current Stimulation

Similar to tDCS, transcranial alternating current stimulation (tACS) applies a weak oscillating electrical current through electrodes placed on the scalp. The current alternates at specific frequencies that aim to synchronize or modulate ongoing brain oscillations. This technique influences cortical excitability by interacting with intrinsic brain rhythms. tACS is being explored for enhancing attention, working memory, and sensorimotor functions by targeting specific neural frequencies.

##### 3.1.4.1.4 Transcranial Random Noise Stimulation

Transcranial random noise stimulation (tRNS) delivers a current composed of random frequencies and amplitudes through scalp electrodes. The stimulation introduces noise to neural circuits, which is believed to enhance signal detection through a process known as stochastic resonance. tRNS has shown promise in improving perceptual learning, motor training, and cognitive performance by modulating cortical excitability in a noninvasive and painless manner.

##### 3.1.4.1.5 Transcranial Focused Ultrasound

Transcranial focused ultrasound (tFUS) uses acoustic waves to modulate brain activity in a targeted and noninvasive manner. A focused ultrasound transducer is placed on the scalp, and low-intensity ultrasound is directed at specific brain regions. The mechanical energy alters neuronal membrane potential, temporarily influencing activity without damaging tissue. tFUS offers high spatial resolution and access to deep brain structures, which is excellent for BCI application and making it a promising technique for future closed-loop systems and targeted neural modulation.

#### 3.1.4.2 Invasive Neural Stimulation

These methods involve surgically implanted electrodes and are mainly used in clinical and high-precision BCI systems for treating neurological disorders or support motor functions.

#### 3.1.4.2.1 *Deep Brain Stimulation*

Deep brain stimulation (DBS) involves implanting electrodes into specific brain regions to deliver controlled electrical stimulation. These electrodes are connected to an implanted pulse generator that sends electrical impulses to modulate the activity of targeted neural circuits. DBS is widely used in the treatment of neurological disorders such as Parkinson's disease and essential tremor. In BCI contexts, DBS can support cognitive or motor functions in clinical populations and represents an example of a fully implantable stimulation system.

### 3.1.4.3 Peripheral and Spinal Stimulation Techniques

Peripheral and spinal stimulation involves the application of electrical or mechanical stimulation to nerves, muscles, or spinal circuits outside the brain to influence motor and sensory pathways. These approaches are often combined with BCI systems for support motor movement and delivering feedback.

#### 3.1.4.3.1 *Functional Electrical Stimulation*

Functional electrical stimulation (FES) delivers electrical impulses to peripheral nerves or muscles to support motor functions. Surface or implanted electrodes stimulate muscles by activating motor neurons, producing contractions that mimic voluntary movement. It is often used in combination with BCIs to enable movement in paralyzed individuals. By interpreting brain signals and translating them into electrical stimulation, FES systems form a crucial component of motor restoration technologies.

#### 3.1.4.3.2 *Peripheral Nerve Stimulation*

Peripheral nerve stimulation (PNS) targets nerves outside the brain and spinal cord, typically through electrodes placed on the skin or implanted near specific nerve bundles. Electrical pulses activate these peripheral nerves, which can restore or enhance motor and sensory functions. In BCI systems, PNS is used to deliver artificial sensory feedback or assist motor output, allowing users to experience more natural and responsive control of prosthetic limbs or exoskeletons.

#### 3.1.4.3.3 *Spinal Cord Stimulation*

Spinal cord stimulation (SCS) delivers electrical impulses to the dorsal columns of the spinal cord through implanted electrodes. The stimulation modifies the transmission of sensory and motor signals along the spinal pathways. SCS is primarily used for managing chronic pain, but in BCI contexts it is being explored for enabling voluntary movement and improving locomotion in individuals with spinal cord injuries. When paired with BCI control, it may help bridge damaged motor pathways to restore functional output.

#### 3.1.4.4 Autonomic Nervous System Modulation

Autonomic Nervous System modulation refers to techniques that regulate physiological functions such as heart rate, respiration, and gastrointestinal activity by influencing the sympathetic and parasympathetic branches of the nervous system.

##### *3.1.4.4.1 Vagus Nerve Stimulation*

Vagus nerve stimulation (VNS) involves delivering mild electrical pulses to the vagus nerve, which connects the brain to multiple internal organs. This stimulation can be administered using implanted electrodes in the neck or through external devices placed on the skin near the ear. VNS modulates brain activity indirectly by influencing brainstem nuclei and promoting widespread cortical changes. VNS is being investigated for enhancing learning and neuroplasticity, particularly in motor rehabilitation and adaptive feedback systems.

#### 3.1.4.5 Tactile Feedback Techniques

These methods deliver feedback to the user through the skin, closing the loop in BCI systems by providing sensory information in response to brain activity.

##### *3.1.4.5.1 Electrotactile and Vibrotactile Feedback*

Electrotactile and vibrotactile feedback techniques deliver stimulation to the skin using small electrical currents or mechanical vibrations. These methods are commonly used in BCIs to provide real-time feedback about system state or user performance. By activating sensory receptors in the skin, they create an artificial sense of touch or pressure, which can be used to convey information from a prosthetic limb, guide motor actions, or improve user engagement in assistive technologies.

### 3.1.5 Emerging and Hybrid Acquisition Techniques

Beyond the established invasive and noninvasive approaches, several emerging and hybrid methods are growing, which aim to bridge the gap between high signal fidelity and practical usability. These innovative techniques leverage advances in materials science, optics, and miniaturized sensors to improve comfort, reduce invasiveness, and enhance recording quality.

#### 3.1.5.1 High-density and Flexible EEG

Recent advances in high-density EEG (HD-EEG) and emerging ultra–HD EEG systems have introduced soft, flexible electrode arrays that significantly enhance spatial resolution and user comfort. Conductive polymers, stretchable substrates, and dry or semidry electrodes enable rapid setup and long-term monitoring, expanding EEG's applicability to wearable and mobile BCIs with high spatial resolution. See example of one such ultra HD-EEG in Figure 3.5.

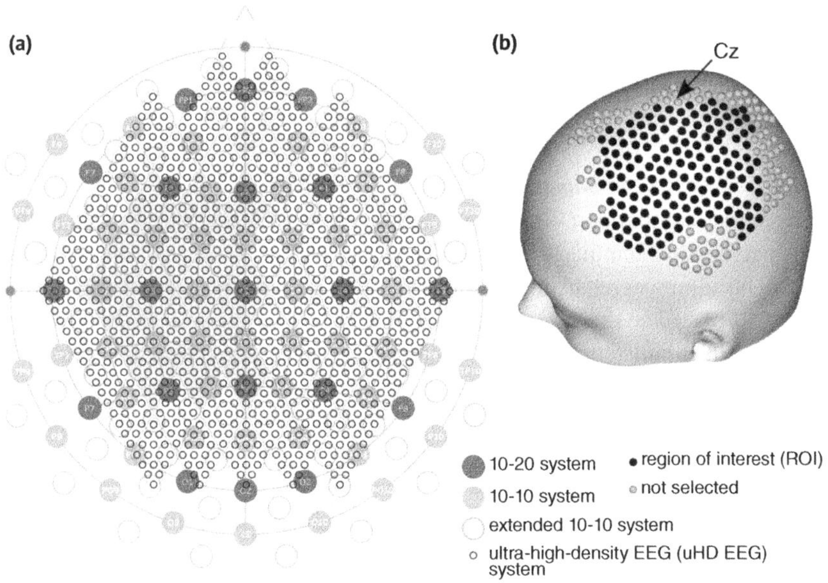


**Figure 3.5** An ultra-high-density electroencephalography (uHD EEG): (a) schematic of uHD EEG system in comparison of standard EEG system including standard electrode placement schemes – 10–20, 10–10, and extended 10–10; (b) a 3D head model with uHD EEG system and a marked electrode positions Cz. *Source*: [57]/Frontiers Media S.A./CC BY 4.0.

#### 3.1.5.2 Portable MEG Using Optically Pumped Magnetometers

Traditional MEG requires large cryogenic systems, but optically pumped magnetometers (OPMs) make it possible for lightweight, room-temperature MEG systems [55]. Although these systems are still experimental, OPM-based MEG allows participants to move freely during recording, opening opportunities for naturalistic BCI applications. Some examples of this system are shown in Figure 3.6.

#### 3.1.5.3 Functional Ultrasound Imaging

Functional ultrasound (fUS) is an emerging modality capable of detecting hemodynamic changes with higher spatial resolution than fNIRS and better portability than fMRI. Early studies suggest its potential for real-time decoding of motor intentions in animal models.

#### 3.1.5.4 Hybrid EEG–fNIRS Systems

Hybrid systems combine complementary modalities, such as EEG and fNIRS, to balance temporal and spatial resolution. These multimodal setups enhance decoding accuracy and robustness, particularly in cognitive state monitoring, mental workload assessment, and low-bandwidth communication BCIs.

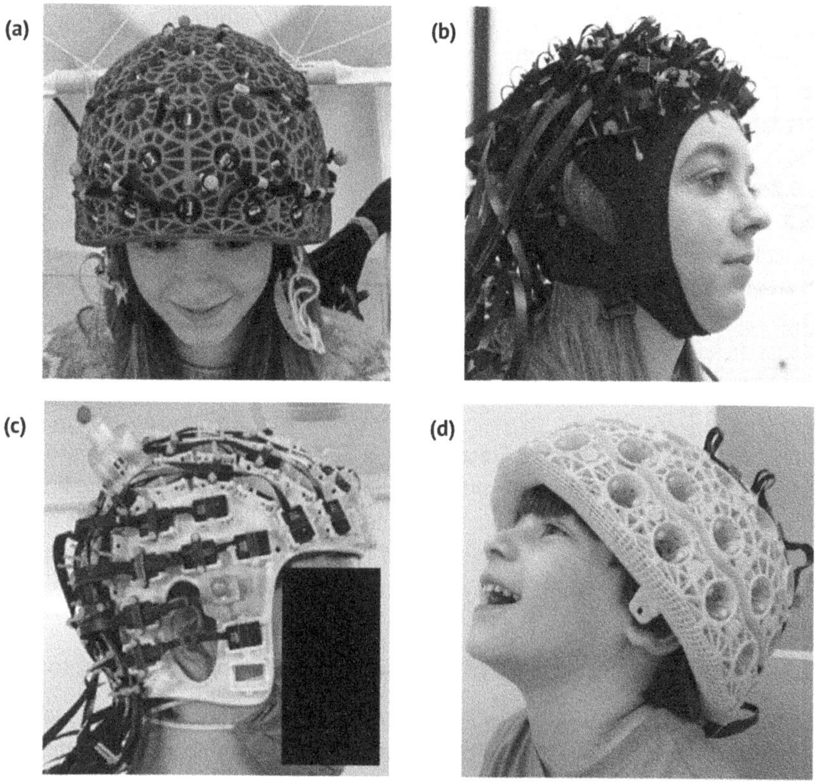


**Figure 3.6** Different OPM–MEG systems in operation within controlled environments. (a) A flexible, lightweight helmet; (b) an EEG-like flexible MEG system; (c) another OPM–MEG design adjustable for different head sizes; (d) a 3D-printed MEG helmet with OPM sensors. *Source*: [58]/Elsevier/CC BY 4.0.

### 3.1.6 Wireless and Minimally Invasive Neural Interfaces

Recent development in devices is also focus on improving the long-term practicality of invasive BCIs by removing percutaneous connectors, reducing surgical burden, and increasing user mobility.

#### 3.1.6.1 Wireless Intracortical Implants

Next-generation intracortical systems integrate wireless power and data transmission to eliminate skin-penetrating connectors. These devices reduce infection risk, improve comfort, and support continuous home-based operation. A prominent example is the Neuralink implant, which embeds flexible polymer electrode threads into the cortex and transmits digitized neural data wirelessly to an external device. By combining high channel count intracortical recording with a fully implantable, sealed, and rechargeable package, systems like Neuralink illustrate the trend toward long-term, unobtrusive neural interfaces suitable for everyday use.

#### 3.1.6.2 Endovascular Recording Systems

The Stentrode which has been discussed before under section "invasive acquisition technologies" represents a new class of minimally invasive neural interface delivered through the vascular system rather than open-brain surgery as well. By deploying electrodes inside cortical blood vessels, these systems capture ECoG-like signals while substantially reducing surgical risk. Their vascular anchoring and wireless telemetry make them strong candidates for long-term clinical use.

#### 3.1.6.3 Soft and Bio-integrated Electronics

Emerging devices made from ultrathin, flexible materials conform to the brain's surface and reduce tissue irritation. These bio-integrated electrodes can be delivered through smaller surgical openings and provide stable, high-density recordings with improved biocompatibility compared to rigid electrodes.

### 3.1.7 Closed-loop Integration of Acquisition and Stimulation Technologies

Acquisition and stimulation technologies increasingly operate together in closed-loop systems that not only sense neural activity and interpret it, but also deliver stimulation in real time. This bidirectional interaction forms the foundation of adaptive BCIs or two-way BCI systems capable of modulating neural circuits based on ongoing physiological states. Closed-loop systems differ fundamentally from their open-loop counterparts by continuously adjusting stimulation parameters according to the user's current neural responses rather than relying on predetermined or fixed settings.

There are several prominent examples that have demonstrated the potential of closed-loop BCIs. Adaptive deep brain stimulation (aDBS) adjusts stimulation intensity based on pathological oscillations detected from implanted electrodes, showing improved outcomes for Parkinson's disease compared to continuous DBS. Brain–spinal interfaces can decode motor intentions from cortical activity and immediately stimulate spinal circuits to restore voluntary movement in individuals with spinal cord injury. Similarly, sensorimotor neuroprostheses integrate high-resolution intracortical recordings with tactile or electrotactile feedback, enabling users to control robotic limbs while perceiving a sense of touch or pressure.

## 3.2 Summary

This chapter has provided an overview of the core technologies that enable the operation of BCI systems. We examined both acquisition technologies, which capture and interpret neural signals, and stimulation technologies, which allow BCIs to influence or interact with the nervous system. Together, these technologies form the foundation of bidirectional communication between the brain and external devices.

Noninvasive acquisition methods such as EEG, fNIRS, and MEG offer accessible and widely used options, while invasive techniques like intracortical electrodes and ECoG provide high-resolution data critical for advanced applications. This chapter also highlighted emerging and hybrid approaches including high-density EEG, portable MEG, functional ultrasound, and multimodal EEG–fNIRS systems as well as new wireless and minimally invasive interfaces like Neuralink and the Stentrode that aim to improve long-term practicality.

Similarly, stimulation technologies range from noninvasive approaches like tDCS and TMS to more invasive interventions such as DBS, peripheral nerve stimulation, and spinal cord stimulation. These tools not only serve therapeutic roles but also support adaptive feedback and enhanced user interaction. With the growing integration of acquisition and stimulation, closed-loop BCI systems are becoming increasingly feasible, enabling responsive, context-aware modulation of neural circuits in real time.

The next chapter will explore how these technologies are applied in specific use cases, from assistive communication systems to neurorehabilitation and cognitive enhancement, demonstrating their impact across healthcare, research, and human–machine interaction.

# 4

# Translational Brain–Computer Interfaces: Bridging Research to Practice

Translational neuroscience focuses on applying discoveries from basic research to the development of clinical applications and treatments for neurological and psychiatric disorders. Acting as a bridge between laboratory research and patient care, it seeks to transform scientific findings into effective diagnostics, therapies, and interventions. Translational brain–computer interface (BCI) expands this concept beyond traditional clinical boundaries. It encompass a broader spectrum of neurotechnology applications, including cognitive enhancement, functional augmentation, entertainment, education, and adaptive human-computer interaction. Translational BCIs aim to leverage neuroscience insights in both medical and non-medical contexts, promoting the integration of neurotechnologies into everyday life. The goal of translational BCI is to take insights and tools developed under controlled experimental conditions and adapt them for meaningful use in real-world environments. This involves addressing key challenges such as usability, robustness, adaptability, and seamless integration into everyday life. This chapter examines how BCI systems progress from theoretical models and lab-based prototypes to practical tools used in real-world settings across medical, rehabilitative, and consumer domains. It also highlights the core principles, challenges, and case studies that define the evolving field of translational BCI.

## 4.1 Clinical and Neuroscientific Foundations of Translational BCI

Mental health research has been a major driving force behind current developments in BCI technology, particularly with the goal of treating or managing conditions such as depression, bipolar disorder, schizophrenia, neurodegenerative diseases, traumatic brain injury, chronic pain, and epilepsy. BCIs have emerged as a promising tool in this domain by enabling the monitoring of neural patterns, providing neurofeedback, and facilitating therapeutic engagement aimed at improving mental well-being. Beyond mental health treatment, BCIs have also found valuable applications in broader clinical and assistive settings. They can offer alternative communication pathways for individuals with spinal cord injuries or severe motor impairments, helping to restore some level of interaction with their environment. These applications highlight the translational potential of BCI technology, making it a versatile solution across different patient populations, healthcare environments, and stages of illness.

### 4.1.1 BCI Contributing to Clinical Research

The foundation of BCI research is based on fundamental understanding of neural mechanisms, not only to drive new technological developments but also to expand our knowledge in clinical contexts such as drug development and diagnostic testing for clinical solution. BCIs contribute to this field by offering real-time access to brain activity, allowing researchers to explore how the brain responds to various pharmacological and therapeutic interventions. For example, in preclinical studies using animal models of depression, BCIs can assist in screening the efficacy of new treatments by providing continuous neural monitoring. In human studies, neural biomarkers captured through electroencephalography (EEG) or functional magnetic resonance imaging (fMRI), integrated with BCI systems, may serve as valuable tools for diagnosing mental health conditions or tracking changes during treatment. These neural markers offer insights into individual responses and help in tailoring more precise interventions.

The translational value of BCI in clinical research depends on its ability to bridge findings from controlled experimental environments to real-world human conditions. Ensuring that results obtained in laboratory settings retain their relevance and reliability in natural clinical contexts is essential for meaningful progress. This ability to connect basic neuroscience with applied medicine places BCIs at the intersection of discovery and treatment.

### 4.1.2 Insights from Cellular Neuroscience

In parallel with clinical research using BCI applications to test and evaluate brain functions, there is a growing interest on imaging and decoding neural activity at the cellular scale. This level of investigation explores how learning, memory, and emotion emerge from the interactions of individual neurons and brain circuits. Insights gained from this cellular-level research contribute not only to our fundamental understanding of the brain but also to the development of new interventions. These range from pharmacological approaches aimed at creating more targeted therapies to more advanced and creative forms of invasive BCI. Research at the cellular scale plays a critical role in shaping how BCIs are designed and how they operate. By understanding the neural dynamics that underlie specific cognitive and emotional processes, this work informs the development of algorithms and intervention strategies that are more precise and responsive. Ultimately, the goal is to enhance or restore brain function in individuals affected by neurological and psychiatric conditions. This level of study forms a foundational layer that supports innovation across both experimental and applied BCI research.

### 4.1.3 BCI Strategies for Cognitive and Behavioral Modulation

Cognitive-level BCIs are focused on developing applications that aim to enhance mental processes often affected by psychiatric disorders. Cognitive-level BCIs are directed toward developing applications that aim to enhance and augment cognitive processes in neurodiverse groups. These BCIs are designed with the understanding of how cognitive functions such as attention, memory, and decision-making operate in the brain. Techniques like brain imaging have contributed to therapeutic strategies such as cognitive behavioral therapy (CBT), which is commonly used by psychiatrists in clinical treatment. In addition, neurofeedback therapy has gained attention as a method that allows individuals to observe and regulate their brain activity, leading to improvements in conditions like depression, attention deficit hyperactivity disorder (ADHD), post-traumatic stress disorder (PTSD), and even more recent areas like phantom pain reduction and memory enhancement.

The insights gained from these cognitive and therapeutic approaches play a key role in shaping the design of BCIs that respond to real-time brain signals. These systems not only track neural activity but also provide meaningful feedback or stimulation to help users manage cognitive symptoms more effectively. Translational BCI research in this area is aimed at supporting users' mental wellbeing by reinforcing healthy brain patterns and promoting adaptive changes, contributing to long-term cognitive stability and mental well-being.

## 4.2 Real-world Deployment of BCI Systems

Cognitive neuroscience research has traditionally taken place in controlled laboratory environments, where isolating specific variables allows researchers to identify clear cause-and-effect relationships. While this approach has generated valuable insights, many of these findings struggle to translate effectively into real-world settings, particularly when applied for diagnostic or therapeutic purposes. One key reason is that natural cognition is dynamic and far more complex than what is typically captured in structured experiments. To address this challenge, researchers have begun shifting toward the study of cognition and behavior in more naturalistic environments, a direction often referred to as the investigation of natural cognition.

### 4.2.1 Mobile Brain and Body Imaging Approaches

Mobile brain and body imaging (MoBI) integrates portable EEG/functional near-infrared spectroscopy (fNIRS) with motion tracking technologies to record both brain activity and physical movement in large lab spaces or semi-controlled environments. This setup enables individuals to walk, gesture, and interact with their surroundings in ways that more closely resemble real-life behavior, while their neural and bodily responses are continuously monitored. MoBI enhances the ecological validity of neural data, allowing researchers to study the brain in action rather than in isolation. For BCI research, this approach is particularly valuable. It supports the development of systems that are robust in natural environments, where noise from movement, shifting attention, and external stimuli would normally interfere with performance. By understanding how cognition unfolds in real-world settings, BCI researchers can design algorithms and interfaces that account for and adapt to these natural fluctuations. A typical MoBI setup can be seen in Figure 4.1.

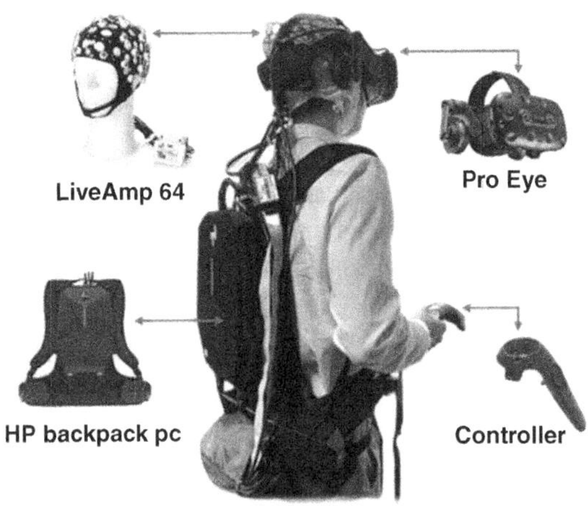


**Figure 4.1** A standard MoBI setup where user is equipped with wireless EEG system with backpack immersed into VR environment and performing task with natural movement while motion also captured via external camera. *Source*: [59]/Springer Nature/CC BY 4.0.

### 4.2.2 Context-aware BCI in Natural Environments

This approach involves deploying sensors and systems in real-world environments like homes, schools, or public spaces. The systems not only collect brain data in real-world but also consider surrounding context such as social cues, environmental stimuli, or user behavior. This supports the development of adaptive BCI that responds to user needs and changing conditions.

## 4.3 Bridging Theory and Application in Translational BCI

For BCI to succeed in practice, it must integrate knowledge from multiple layers of neuroscience as discussed in the previous section. Signals recorded at the cellular level inform decoding algorithms. Cognitive models guide how the interface interacts with the user. Whereas clinical insights shape the goals and constraints of design. Therefore, translational BCI bridges the foundational knowledge of brain mechanics that gradually evolve into functional technologies with direct human applications for communication, rehabilitation, learning, and human–machine interaction. This following case study connects all these dots to bridge theory into real-world BCI applications.

### 4.3.1 SSVEP for Robot Control

#### 4.3.1.1 Fundamental Understanding

Steady-state Visually Evoked Potentials (SSVEPs) are rhythmic electrical responses generated in the visual cortex when a person fixates on a visual stimulus that flickers at a constant frequency. These responses are most prominent in the occipital region of the brain and can be detected using EEG. The key property of SSVEP is that the frequency of the brain's response matches the frequency of the visual stimulus, allowing researchers to identify the stimulus a person is attending to based on the frequency components of the EEG signal. Unlike other brain responses, SSVEPs are sustained over time and produce clear, periodic patterns that are highly stable across trials and individuals. This makes them especially suitable for BCI systems that require high signal reliability and minimal training.

#### 4.3.1.2 Methods and System Design

SSVEP-based BCI systems typically involve a visual interface that displays multiple targets, each flickering at a different frequency. These targets may be represented as boxes, symbols, or directional arrows on a computer screen or tablet. When the user focuses their gaze on a specific flickering target, the visual cortex becomes entrained to the frequency of that stimulus, and this entrainment is reflected in the EEG signal. The system captures real-time EEG data from electrodes placed on the scalp, usually around the occipital area. Signal processing techniques such as Fourier analysis or canonical correlation analysis are then used to identify the dominant frequency in the EEG. Once the system detects which frequency is most prominent, it maps that frequency to the corresponding command.

In a robotic assistance arm interface as shown in Figure 4.2a, each potential options, for example, move hand to pick water, feed different food items, or go back to different options can linked to a target flickering at a unique frequency. When the user looks at the "Water" stimulus, their EEG reflects the associated frequency, and the BCI interprets this as a command to move robot to pick up water and provide to use. The entire process occurs in near real time, usually with minimal delay. Because SSVEP signals do not require the user to learn or train over long sessions, the system can be used by beginners and adapted quickly across different users. Most setups use commercially available EEG devices with 8–32 channels, making these systems relatively cost-effective and portable. Figure 4.2 shows an example where SSVEP was used to demonstrate eating assistance system [60].

#### 4.3.1.3 Application in Real World

In real-world environments, SSVEP-based BCIs are being used in assistive and interactive technologies designed to enhance autonomy for individuals with motor impairments. One of the most impactful applications is robotic wheelchair control. Users with conditions such as spinal cord injury, cerebral palsy, or muscular dystrophy can navigate their surroundings independently by visually selecting movement directions. These systems have been tested in indoor and semi-structured outdoor environments and have shown high accuracy and safety when properly calibrated. Beyond mobility, SSVEP BCIs are also applied to control robotic manipulators, allowing users to perform simple object interaction tasks, such as picking up items, pressing buttons, or moving tools. In some setups, drones have been controlled via SSVEP by mapping altitude, directional movement, and takeoff or landing commands to specific visual frequencies. These systems open new possibilities for exploration, inspection, or personal use, especially in situations where conventional manual control is not possible.

In the context of smart environments, SSVEP systems can be designed to control household appliances. For instance, lights, fans, thermostats, and entertainment systems can be switched on or off using gaze-controlled interfaces. This can significantly improve the quality of life for individuals with severe disabilities, allowing for greater independence in their homes without relying on voice commands or physical touch.

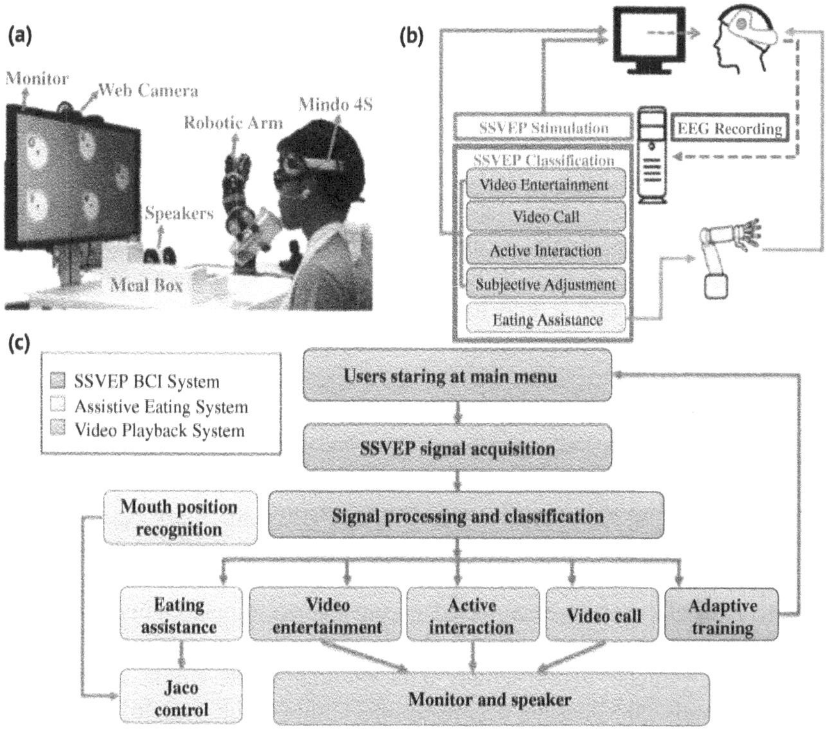


**Figure 4.2** Wireless multifunctional SSVEP-based BCI assistive eating system. (a) System setup which include a computer host, a wireless EEG cap (Mindo 4S), a robotic arm, a set of speakers, a meal box, a high refresh rate monitor and a Web camera. *Source*: [60]/with permission of IEEE. (b) The computer host sends the SSVEP stimulation command to the monitor and collects the EEG data recorded by Mindo 4S via Bluetooth transmission. It then executes SSVEP classification and sends the command to the corresponding subsystem to complete the task. *Source*: [60]/with permission of IEEE. (c) Block diagram of the integrated assistive eating system. The SSVEP BCI system transforms the user's EEG signal into commands and triggers the selected service of the two subsystems, the assistive eating system and the video playback system. A subjective training option is also included in this system to optimally adjust the model for the current user in a short training period. *Source*: [60]/with permission of IEEE.

## 4.3.2 Deep Brain Stimulation for Parkinson's Disease

### 4.3.2.1 Fundamental Understanding

Research into the brain's motor control systems, particularly the role of the basal ganglia, has provided critical insights into the mechanisms behind voluntary movement. The basal ganglia form a complex network with the cortex and thalamus, regulating the initiation and smooth execution of motor commands. In

Parkinson's disease, degeneration of dopamine-producing neurons in the substantia nigra disrupts this circuit, leading to excessive activity in some regions and reduced activity in others. These shifts create imbalances that interfere with normal motor function. As a result, patients experience symptoms such as tremor at rest, muscular rigidity, postural instability, and slowed movement. Over time, these symptoms become increasingly resistant to pharmacological treatments. Through detailed neural recordings and clinical observation, researchers identified specific firing patterns and oscillatory activity in the subthalamic nucleus and globus pallidus that correlate with the severity of these motor impairments. Understanding this pathological activity has laid the foundation for developing targeted neural interventions.

#### 4.3.2.2 Methods and Technological Development

Deep brain stimulation (DBS) emerged as a method to directly modulate abnormal brain activity through precisely delivered electrical stimulation. The technique involves implanting electrodes into deep brain structures known to be involved in the dysregulated motor circuits of Parkinson's disease. The most common targets are the subthalamic nucleus and the internal segment of the globus pallidus. Once implanted, the electrodes are connected to a pulse generator placed under the skin near the chest, as shown in Figure 4.3. This device continuously delivers electrical impulses that influence neural activity at the stimulation site. Unlike lesion-based surgical methods, DBS does not negatively affect brain tissue. Instead, it alters the firing dynamics of neurons in a way that disrupts pathological patterns and facilitates more normal signaling within the motor pathways.

The parameters of stimulation, such as frequency, amplitude, and pulse width, are not fixed. They can be adjusted over time based on the patient's clinical response. This adaptability allows clinicians to fine-tune the system to minimize side effects while maximizing therapeutic benefits. More recent advancements include the development of closed-loop DBS systems, which monitor brain signals in real time and dynamically adjust stimulation in response to changes in neural activity. These systems aim to provide more efficient symptom control and reduce the need for frequent manual reprogramming.

#### 4.3.2.3 Application in Real World

DBS has moved from a novel neurosurgical technique to a well-established therapeutic option for individuals with advanced Parkinson's disease. For many patients whose symptoms are no longer manageable with medication alone, DBS offers significant improvement in daily functioning. After surgery, patients typically go through a period of post-operative programming, where clinicians gradually identify the most effective stimulation settings. This process involves both objective

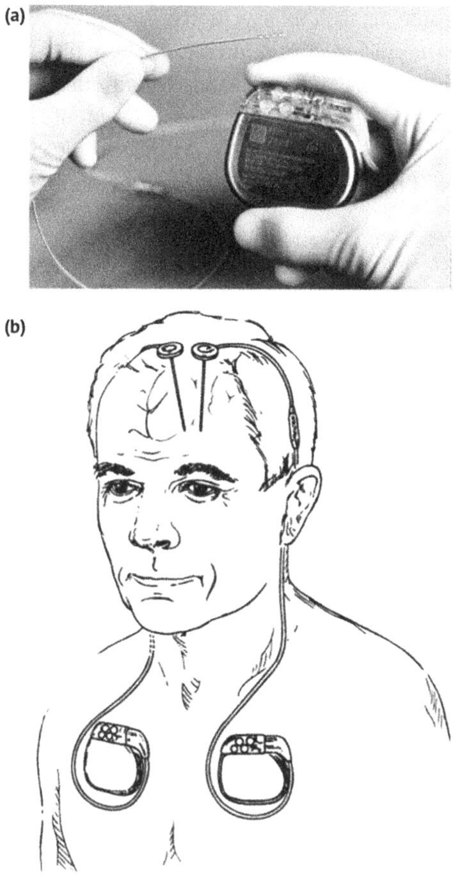


**Figure 4.3** (a) The DBS system. The system consists of a pulse generator (pacemaker) an extension and a brain electrode with four contacts; and (b) bilateral DBS systems in place. *Source*: [61]/with permission of Elsevier.

motor assessments and feedback from the individual about changes in tremor control, coordination, and quality of life. In daily life, patients with DBS often experience reduced tremor, increased fluidity of movement, and more stable posture. This allows them to perform activities such as walking, eating, dressing, or writing with greater ease. Many patients are also able to reduce their reliance on medication, which can help lessen side effects like dyskinesia or nausea. Long-term studies have shown that DBS can maintain its benefits for many years, although continued follow-up and periodic adjustments are typically required.

DBS has also expanded beyond Parkinson's disease, with research and clinical trials exploring its use in other movement disorders such as dystonia and essential tremor, like Locked-in-Syndrome, as well as psychiatric conditions like obsessive-compulsive disorder and treatment-resistant depression. These broader applications reflect the strength of the underlying approach, which combines neuroscience-based targeting with engineering innovation. The evolution of DBS from foundational studies on basal ganglia dysfunction to a widely accessible clinical tool demonstrate the full trajectory of translational neuroscience in action.

### 4.3.3 BCI for Paralysis

#### 4.3.3.1 Fundamental Understanding

In individuals with paralysis, the connection between the brain and the body is disrupted, often due to spinal cord injury, stroke, or neurodegenerative disease. However, research has consistently shown that motor intention such that an act of planning or imagining a movement remains intact in many of these individuals. The motor cortex, which is responsible for generating movement-related signals, continues to exhibit activity even when the corresponding muscles do not respond. These neural patterns, often referred to as movement-related potentials or sensorimotor rhythms, provide a critical entry point for BCI systems. Studies using functional neuroimaging and electrophysiological recordings have revealed that specific regions of the brain activate in predictable ways during both actual and imagined movement. This has led to the understanding that voluntary motor commands can still be accessed directly from the brain, even in the absence of muscle activity. The ability to detect and interpret these brain signals forms the core scientific basis for BCIs aimed at restoring function in individuals with paralysis.

#### 4.3.3.2 Signal Acquisition and Processing Methods

To access motor-related brain activity, BCI systems use either noninvasive or invasive recording techniques. Noninvasive methods such as EEG are widely used due to their safety and accessibility. EEG systems place electrodes on the scalp to record electrical activity generated by cortical neurons. While the spatial resolution is limited, EEG remains effective for capturing broad patterns related to motor intention, particularly in the sensorimotor areas. However, for precise and robust signal acquisition, invasive methods are commonly used as well. Electrocorticography (ECoG) involves placing electrodes directly on the surface of the brain, providing better spatial resolution and signal stability. In some advanced systems, microelectrode arrays are implanted into the motor cortex to record activity from individual neurons. These high-resolution signals allow for fine control, which is especially useful in applications involving multi-joint or dexterous movements.

Once the signals are acquired, they are processed using machine learning algorithms. These algorithms are trained to recognize patterns associated with motor intentions, such as reaching, grasping, or directional movement. The system then converts these patterns into control commands in real time, enabling users to manipulate devices with thought alone. Continuous feedback and adaptive algorithms improve performance over time, allowing the BCI to become more responsive to the user's intentions and cognitive state. Figure 4.4 shows an example BCI based on invasive ECoG to enable movement in patient with quadriplegia [62].

#### 4.3.3.3 Application in Real World

BCI systems for individuals with paralysis have moved beyond proof-of-concept studies and are now being used in various real-world scenarios. In clinical and home settings, users have been able to communicate through screen-based interfaces by selecting letters or icons with their brain signals. These systems often use virtual keyboards where the user navigates a cursor or highlights selections with brain signals, providing an essential communication tool for individuals with locked-in syndrome or advanced amyotrophic lateral sclerosis (ALS). In more advanced applications, BCIs have been used to control robotic limbs and prosthetic devices. For example, users have successfully grasped and moved objects with robotic arms driven entirely by brain activity. These systems interpret motor intentions in real time, allowing for fluid and intuitive control. In some cases, sensory feedback from the device is integrated back into the user's brain through stimulation, closing the loop and restoring a sense of touch.

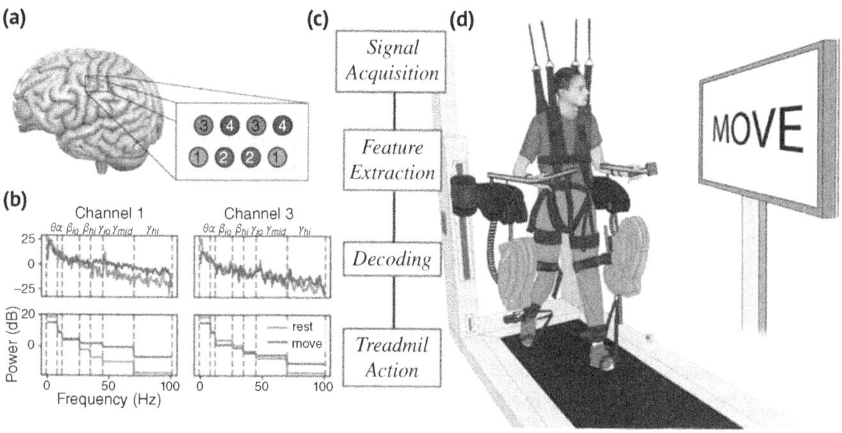


**Figure 4.4** Experimental setup for BCI-controlled ReoAmbulator [62]. (a) Two four channel electrode in sensorimotor cortex related with hand. *Source*: [62]/Frontiers Media S.A./CC BY 4.0. (b) Mean spectral power of select frequency bins for each trial from four electrodes to be used for decoder training and testing. *Source*: [62]/Frontiers Media S.A./CC BY 4.0. (c) Signal processing pipeline used in ReoAmbulator. *Source*: [62]/Frontiers Media S.A./CC BY 4.0. (d) Stimulus shows to used for motor imagery task on a large display while acquiring brain signals. *Source*: [62]/Frontiers Media S.A./CC BY 4.0.

Wearable exoskeletons represent another area of practical application. Individuals with lower-limb paralysis have been able to initiate walking or standing by imagining the movement, with the BCI system translating this intention into action through robotic support. These systems not only provide mobility but also offer psychological and physiological benefits by enabling upright posture and physical activity. Despite these achievements, challenges remain in making BCIs fully practical for everyday use. Variability in signal quality across sessions, the need for extensive training, and system calibration are ongoing barriers. Environmental factors, user fatigue, and changes in attention can also affect performance. To address these challenges, current research is focused on developing adaptive systems that can learn from the user, minimize calibration time, and operate reliably across different contexts.

### 4.3.4 High-bandwidth Speech Restoration

#### 4.3.4.1 Fundamental Understanding

Speech production relies on coordinated neural activity in the ventral motor cortex, premotor cortex, and language-associated regions such as Broca's area. Even in individuals with conditions such as ALS or brainstem stroke, the neural representations of intended speech often remain preserved despite loss of muscle control. Research over the past decade has shown that high-channel-count intracortical recordings can capture detailed neural firing patterns associated with attempted speech movements, including phoneme- and syllable-level representations. This provides the scientific foundation for developing BCIs that decode intended speech directly from cortical activity.

#### 4.3.4.2 Methods and System Design

Paradromics' *Connexus* system is an invasive BCI designed specifically for speech restoration. The implant uses a high-density array of approximately 420 microwire electrodes that penetrate the cortical surface and record activity from populations of neurons involved in the articulation of speech. Neural signals are acquired, digitized, and wirelessly transmitted to an external computer, where machine learning models decode the user's intended speech in real time. The system is fully implantable, designed for long-term use, and aims to support communication speeds approaching natural typing rates. Algorithms trained on neural activity during attempted speech map firing patterns onto letters, words, or synthesized speech outputs.

#### 4.3.4.3 Application in Real World

In 2025, Paradromics received Food and Drug Administration (FDA) approval to begin the first long-term human trial of the Connexus implant as shown in

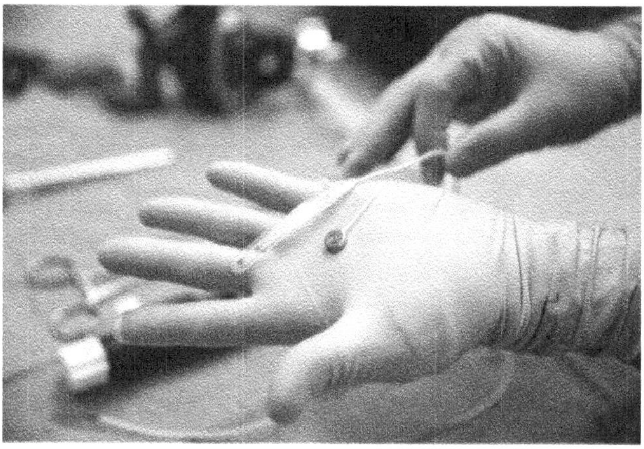

The Regents of the University of Michigan Health

**Figure 4.5** The paradromics connexus high-bandwidth BCI implant: cortical module and wireless transceiver system.

Figure 4.5, marking a significant milestone in translational BCI. The system is being tested in individuals with severe motor impairments who are unable to communicate verbally. Early surgical demonstrations have shown that the device can reliably record high-quality neural data, validating its design for chronic use. If successful, Connexus could provide an intuitive, high-speed communication pathway for individuals with ALS, brainstem stroke, or locked-in conditions, representing a major step forward in accessible neural speech prostheses.

## 4.3.5 Closed-loop Stroke Rehabilitation Using the ReHand-BCI System

### 4.3.5.1 Fundamental Understanding

Stroke often disrupts motor pathways controlling the upper extremities, but residual cortical activity related to movement intention frequently remains intact. Studies in motor imagery and neuroplasticity have demonstrated that pairing voluntary intent with sensory or motor feedback strengthens functional neural connections. This forms the basis for BCI-assisted rehabilitation: detecting motor-related brain signals and linking them to robotic assistance to reinforce appropriate neural pathways.

### 4.3.5.2 Methods and System Design

The ReHand-BCI platform [63] combines EEG-based detection of motor imagery with a robotic hand orthosis (Figure 4.6). During training sessions, patients attempt or imagine hand movements while EEG sensors capture corresponding cortical activity. When the system detects appropriate neural patterns, it triggers the robotic orthosis to perform the intended movement, providing real-time visual

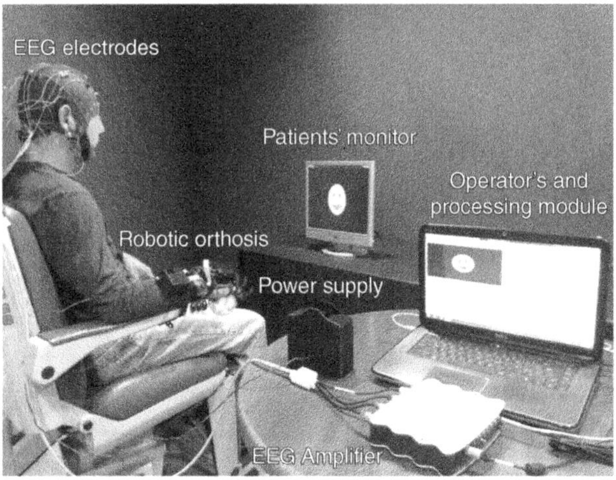


**Figure 4.6** The ReHand-BCI system combining EEG-based motor imagery decoding with a robotic hand orthosis for stroke upper-limb rehabilitation. *Source*: [63]/Frontiers Media S.A./CC BY 4.0.

and proprioceptive feedback. A randomized controlled trial compared this closed-loop BCI-assisted therapy against a sham-BCI control condition, with both groups participating in structured rehabilitation sessions.

#### 4.3.5.3 Application in Real World

Results from the clinical trial showed that patients using the active BCI system demonstrated greater improvements in upper-limb motor function compared to control participants, as measured by commonly used assessment tools such as the Fugl–Meyer (FMA-UE) scale. Neurophysiological markers indicated enhanced cortical reorganization, suggesting that closed-loop BCI therapy can accelerate post-stroke recovery. The ReHand-BCI system represents a promising translational example in neurorehabilitation and may become part of clinical protocols for restoring hand function after stroke.

## 4.4 Summary

Translational BCI represents a convergence of basic neuroscience, engineering innovation, and real-world human needs. By extending beyond the restricted and controlled laboratory studies, BCI technologies are increasingly demonstrating their potential across medical, rehabilitative, educational, and assistive domains. From neural signal decoding at the cellular level to adaptive applications in natural environments, the field continues to evolve toward systems that are both scientifically grounded and practically usable. Clinical applications have already begun to reshape how we approach conditions such as paralysis, Parkinson's disease, and mood disorders, offering new avenues for communication, mobility, and cognitive rehabilitation. At the same time, advances in mobile sensing, real-time feedback, and context-aware computing are enabling BCIs to function reliably in the complexity of everyday life. These developments reflect a shift from proof-of-concept systems to meaningful tools that can integrate seamlessly with users' goals and environments. Translational success requires sustained collaboration across disciplines, as well as a commitment to addressing challenges related to usability, personalization, and long-term engagement. As BCI systems become more adaptive, intelligent, and user-centric, they open the door not only to treatment but also to augmentation, learning, and personal empowerment. The future of translational BCI lies in continuing to bridge science and society, ensuring that innovations in brain technology lead to tangible improvements in quality of life.

# 5

# Automated Signal Processing for Neural Interfaces

Artificial intelligence (AI) has shown significant progress in the past decade, with a trend toward a rise in sophisticated machine learning (ML) models, including a steady progress in large foundational models like large language models (LLMs) and large vision models (LVMs). Neural interfaces with brain-computer interfaces (BCIs), as a primary example, are significantly dependent on ML for preprocessing, accurate decoding, and prediction. This reliance becomes even more critical in real-world environments, where BCIs must process multimodal data under dynamic and often unpredictable conditions. As users operate in complex, noisy, and constantly changing settings involving shifting attention, physical movement, and diverse environmental contexts, neural interface decoding systems must be accurate, adaptive, context-aware, and capable of functioning in real time with high accuracy. The continued advancement of neural interface technology, combined with improvements in both signal acquisition hardware and intelligent AI systems, is opening new frontiers in human–computer interaction, cognitive augmentation, and assistive technologies.

This chapter provides a comprehensive overview of the automated signal processing approaches used in BCI research and practice. It covers traditional signal processing techniques, automated and adaptive pipelines, feature extraction methods, nonlinear measures, AI-powered denoising, multimodal considerations, and widely used software tools.

## 5.1 From Traditional to Automated Signal Processing

Signal processing is an essential part of BCIs, which provide all necessary methods required to extract and interpret neural data. These methods are built up over time as the field progresses and are highly dependent on manual processes and expert knowledge which is acceptable for offline data analysis for data collected in a controlled laboratory environment. However, these methods often struggle with more dynamic and real-world environments, commonly a case of BCIs. Let's explore these common techniques.

## 5.2 Preprocessing and Artifact Handling

### 5.2.1 Preprocessing Techniques

Preprocessing is the crucial step in preparing raw neural data, such as electroencephalography (EEG) for analysis. These signals are commonly contaminated with artifacts from various sources, such as ocular movements, muscle activity, and surrounding electrical noise. To improve signal quality, data has to go through preprocessing steps to prepare it for advanced analysis. An effective preprocessing can significantly improve the signal-to-noise ratio (SNR) and therefore improve the interpretability of signals, along with feature extraction and classification for BCI applications. As the field evolves, preprocessing is becoming more robust and accessible through automated tools and standardized pipelines, streamlining the transition from raw signals to actionable insights. Let's look at the most commonly used preprocessing techniques:

#### 5.2.1.1 Bandpass and Notch Filtering

Bandpass filtering is a crucial preprocessing step in signal analysis, especially for BCI-related acquisition methods such as EEG. The primary goal of any filtering approach is to isolate neural oscillations within specific frequency ranges relevant to cognitive, motor, and sensory functions. In EEG-based BCIs, frequencies below approximately 0.5–1 Hz are typically removed to eliminate baseline drifts caused by perspiration or slow movements, while frequencies above 50–60 Hz are excluded to suppress high-frequency noise such as electromyographic activity and electrical line interference. Several techniques are available for bandpass filtering, with some of the most commonly used including (also see Table 5.1 and visual comparison in Figure 5.1):

- *Finite Impulse Response (FIR) Filtering:* It is known for its linear phase response and stability. It is widely used in offline EEG analysis. FIR filtering minimizes signal distortion; however, it requires high computational resources due to longer filter lengths.
- *Infinite Impulse Response (IIR) Filtering:* It offers faster computation with fewer coefficients, making it suitable for real-time signal processing. However, IIR filtering can introduce phase distortions and is therefore less suitable for applications that rely on phase information.
- *Wavelet-based Filtering:* It allows multiscale signal analysis by decomposing them into time and frequency-based components. This technique is very

effective for nonstationary signals like EEG. It also offers high-resolution detection of transient features but is sensitive to parameter selection and can be computationally complex.

- *Notch Filtering:* It removes narrowband interference, commonly at 50 or 60 Hz, caused by power line artifacts. It is a simple and effective method for eliminating fixed-frequency noise but may risk attenuating nearby useful frequency components.

#### 5.2.1.2 Resampling and Downsampling

Resampling of the data is one of the most common preprocessing steps, which is utilized to adjust the sampling rate of recorded neural data across different modalities, including EEG, magnetoencephalography (MEG), functional near-infrared spectroscopy (fNIRS), electrocorticography (ECoG), and local field potentials (LFPs). Downsampling is one of the resampling approaches where the sampling rate of the original signals is reduced while preserving essential neural information. Both resampling and downsampling are essential steps to standardize data across different data recording setups and configurations as well as to support reducing computational needs. Conversely, upsampling can be used to synchronize data streams across modalities with differing sampling rates.

Before downsampling, anti-aliasing low-pass filtering is required to prevent high-frequency components from folding into lower frequencies. Newer sampling methods employ a variety of techniques for sampling to maintain signal quality

**Table 5.1** Bandpass filtering techniques.

| Filtering method | Key advantages | Limitations | Best use case |
|---|---|---|---|
| **Finite impulse response (FIR)** | • Linear phase response (preserves waveform shape)<br>• Guaranteed stability | • Requires longer filter lengths<br>• High computational load | Offline EEG analysis where accuracy is prioritized over speed |
| **Infinite impulse response (IIR)** | • Computationally efficient<br>• Shorter filter lengths | • May introduce phase distortion<br>• Less stable under certain conditions | Real-time processing where low latency is critical |
| **Wavelet-based filtering** | • Multiscale (time-frequency) analysis<br>• Good for nonstationary/transient features | • Sensitive to parameter tuning<br>• Computationally intensive | Detection of transient or time-varying EEG events |
| **Notch filtering** | • Effectively removes narrowband noise (e.g., 50/60 Hz) | • May attenuate nearby useful frequencies | Eliminating power line interference or other fixed-frequency noise |

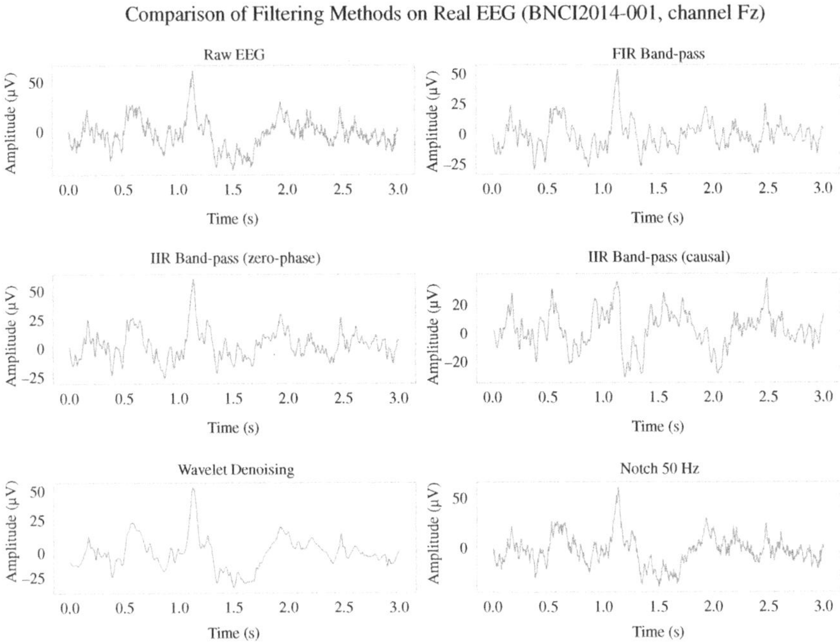


**Figure 5.1** Different filtering techniques applied on raw EEG signals based on BNCI database. *Source*: [64]/Frontiers Media S.A./CC BY 3.0.

and integrity, including interpolation, decimation, and polyphase. A good sampling technique is not just helpful to improve the cross-subject analysis but also supports reproducibility and compatibility with ML and real-time BCI paradigms.

#### 5.2.1.3 DC Offset and Baseline Correction

Direct current (DC) offset refers to a constant shift of the signal away from zero, caused by factors such as electrode polarization, amplifier imbalance, sensor drift, or changes in skin-electrode impedance. This phenomenon is well known to non-invasive techniques like EEG but also present in invasive methods such as ECoG and LFPs due to electrode–tissue interactions and long-term drift. Although DC components do not carry meaningful neural information, they can adversely influence filtering, component decomposition, and algorithms sensitive to baseline fluctuations.

Baseline correction techniques such as mean subtraction, high-pass filtering (typically at 0.1–1 Hz), or polynomial detrending are commonly used to remove DC offsets. These methods help stabilize the signal baseline, prevent numerical issues, and improve the reliability of spectral analysis and feature extraction, particularly in applications requiring consistent amplitude and phase characteristics.

#### 5.2.1.4 Artifact Removal

BCI signals are often contaminated by non-neural artifacts arising from eye movements, blinking, jaw clenching, heartbeat activity, and environmental electromagnetic interference. It is essential to remove these artifacts before further signal processing to improve the signal-to-noise ratio (SNR). Several manual, semi-automatic, and automatic methods have been proposed. Common state-of-the-art techniques for artifact removal include:

##### *5.2.1.4.1 Independent Component Analysis*

Independent component analysis (ICA) is one of the most widely used techniques for artifact removal in EEG and MEG. ICA works by decomposing multichannel signals into a set of statistically independent components (ICs). These ICs could be a mix of distinct sources such as eye saccades, blinks, and muscle artifacts, including genuine brain activity. Based on different properties of these ICs such as topography, power spectrum, and temporal characteristics, artifacts or non-brain sources can be removed to get clean brain-only signals with high SNR. Although ICA is very effective, it still comes with several limitations:

- It assumes that source signals are spatially stationary and independent, which may not be true in all brain recording scenarios.
- It is sensitive to the number of channels and the quality of the data.
- It typically requires a sufficient amount of data (several minutes) to perform reliable component decomposition.
- Real-time implementation is challenging due to computational demands and the need for component classification.

##### *5.2.1.4.2 Principal Component Analysis*

Principal component analysis (PCA) is a dimensionality reduction technique that transforms multichannel data such as EEG into a new set of orthogonal components ranked by the amount of variance they explain in the data. While PCA is useful for noise reduction and feature extraction, it assumes linearity and Gaussianity, making it less effective than ICA for separating biologically meaningful sources or non-Gaussian artifacts. For example, in EEG preprocessing, PCA is sometimes used as a preliminary step to reduce the dimensionality before applying ICA or as a simpler alternative when computational resources are limited. However, since PCA focuses on variance rather than independence, it may retain artifacts if those artifacts dominate the variance in the data. Its main strengths lie in reducing computational load for downstream tasks, highlighting dominant patterns in data, and improving SNR in the signals. However, its limited ability to differentiate artifacts from neural signals restricts its utility in artifact rejection.

#### 5.2.1.4.3 Automatic Subspace Reconstruction

Automatic subspace reconstruction (ASR) is a data-driven method developed for real-time and mobile EEG applications [65]. Although ASR, in principle, can be applied to other continuous neural recordings such as MEG, ECoG, or LFPs, its practical use remains largely limited to EEG. ASR detects and suppresses artifacts by comparing the covariance structure of incoming EEG segments to a clean reference covariance matrix, typically built from artifact-free data. ASR operates by identifying segments that deviate significantly from this baseline, e.g., during motion or muscle spikes, and then reconstructing these using a lower-dimensional subspace that better matches the clean data distribution. This allows ASR to preserve the underlying neural activity while removing transient, high-amplitude artifacts. ASR has significant advantages in real-time compatibility, automatic operation with minimal user input, and high tolerance for noisy, nonstationary data.

However, ASR is sensitive to parameter settings such as thresholding and the quality of the reference data. Improper setting up these parameters can lead to the unintentional removal of valid neural signals or inadequate artifact suppression.

#### 5.2.1.4.4 Regression-based Correction

Regression-based artifact correction methods are based on the relationship between neural recordings such as EEG, MEG, or fNIRS with auxiliary reference channels. These auxiliary channels are used to capture specific sources of contamination, such as electrooculogram (EOG) signals for ocular artifacts or electromyogram (EMG) signals for muscle activity. A regression model is fitted to estimate the contribution of the artifact source to each neural channel, and this estimated component is subsequently subtracted to obtain a cleaned signal. This approach is particularly effective when high-quality reference sensors are available and when the artifacts exhibit consistent temporal or spatial patterns. It has been widely applied in contexts such as eye-movement and blink correction in EEG, motion artifact mitigation in fNIRS, and dual-modality setups where dedicated auxiliary sensors provide reliable artifact measurements.

Although regression-based correction has a number of benefits, it also has several limitations. One such limitation is the assumption of a linear relationship between the reference channel and the contaminated neural signal, which is not always true for nonlinear artifacts. Additionally, the method's effectiveness depends on the quality of reference sensors and the position of auxiliary channels. A poorly aligned sensor can lead to incomplete or inaccurate artifact removal. Moreover, due to regression-based approaches' dependence on the availability of suitable reference channels, they cannot address artifacts for which no corresponding auxiliary channel exists.

##### 5.2.1.4.5 Machine and Deep Learning-based Preprocessing Approaches

Beyond traditional preprocessing, ML and deep learning methods can substantially improve neural data quality by suppressing artifacts. These methods are data-driven, where models learn the structure of both neural signals and artifacts, therefore enabling adaptive and automated preprocessing. For example, hybrid ML pipelines [67] can be used where canonical correlation analysis (CCA) is used to separate autocorrelated neural and nonneural components, followed by probabilistic clustering methods to automatically identify and remove artifact-dominated sources. Such approaches are very useful for real-time suppression of different artifacts, including eye blinks, muscle activity, and movement noise, while preserving the temporal and spectral characteristics of the underlying neural signals.

Deep learning can further enabled end-to-end denoising signal processing that operate directly on raw or minimally processed signals. Neural networks [67] can be trained to map contaminated EEG to artifact-free representations, either through supervised learning or through adaptive online training using auxiliary reference channels. These models can learn complex nonlinear relationships between noise sources and neural activity, supporting robust removal of nonstationary or subject-specific artifacts that are difficult to model using conventional techniques. In particular, real-time deep learning based artifacts removal methods have demonstrated that sample-by-sample adaptation can effectively track and cancel artifacts as they evolve, offering substantial improvements in SNR.

The advantages of machine and deep learning approaches include high automation, strong adaptability to varying recording conditions, and the ability to model intricate spatial–temporal patterns in the data. At the same time, these methods also introduce a number of challenges, such as the need for relevant training data, risks of inadvertently attenuating neural components, and the computational demands associated with real-time deployment.

#### 5.2.1.5 Normalization and Standardization

Normalization is applied to standardize neural signal amplitudes, reducing variability caused by differences in hardware, recording sessions, or subjects. This step particularly important for the robustness and generalizability of statistical and ML models. normalization is optional step in signal processing however it plays an essential role in many pipelines. Some key normalization techniques include:

- *Z-score Normalization:* Standardizes each channel by subtracting its mean and dividing by its standard deviation. By doing so, these normalization techniques help to reduce variability across trials within sessions and subjects. However, at the same time, they could affect the individual differences in neural activity.

- *Min-max Scaling:* Rescales signals to a specific interval, typically between zero and one or between negative one and one. This method is useful for models sensitive to scale but also sensitive to outliers and not robust in non-stationary datasets.
- *Baseline Correction:* Subtracts the average amplitude during a predefined pre-stimulus window to correct for inter-trial and inter-subject variability. This normalization is very common while analyzing data such as EEG, however sensitive to chosen baseline intervals.
- *Quantile Normalization:* Adjusts the distribution of signal amplitudes across trials or subjects to match a reference distribution. This technique is effective in multi-subject studies but may suppress physiologically meaningful differences.
- *Channel-wise Standardization:* Normalizes each EEG channel independently to ensure equal contribution to ML models. This method is useful but may ignore interchannel relationships that are informative for decoding.

## 5.3 Feature Extraction for Neural Interfaces

Once the data have been preprocessed, the next step involves extracting features that encapsulate relevant information from the signal. Feature extraction transforms the high-dimensional time series data into a compact set of descriptors that are informative for classification or regression tasks. These features can be derived from multiple domains such as time, frequency, spatial, and non-linear domains. Time-domain features include statistical moments, amplitude variance, or event-related potentials (ERPs) associated with specific tasks or stimuli. Frequency-domain features are often based on power spectral density (PSD), which reveals the strength of rhythmic activity across different bands such as alpha, beta, or gamma. Spatial features capture the distribution of activity across the scalp or cortical surface and may involve spatial filtering techniques like common spatial patterns (CSPs) or source reconstruction methods. Nonlinear features such as entropy and fractal measures capture signal complexity. These extracted features could be used as input feature for the ML models for decoding and classification in BCI systems.

### 5.3.1 Time-domain Features

Time-domain features operate directly on the raw or preprocessed signal waveforms, extracting simple and informative descriptors such as mean, variance, standard deviation, skewness, kurtosis, and peak-to-peak amplitude. These features are particularly useful in EEG and ECoG data, because they offer high temporal resolution and are sensitive to transient changes such as ERPs. In modalities with slower temporal dynamics like fNIRS or fMRI, time-domain features can still be used but often reflect hemodynamic response patterns rather than electrical transients. These features are popular due in BCIs due to limited computational needs and real-time compatibility. Time-domain features are also easy to interpret, especially with BCI paradigms relevant to strong temporal markers. However, at the same time, these features are highly susceptible to artifacts and may fail to capture underlying spectral or spatial dynamics, limiting their effectiveness when used in isolation. Common feature extraction techniques in the time domain are:

- *Mean and Median:* This is perhaps the most commonly used technique among researchers. These basic measures of central tendency capture the average or typical signal amplitude over a defined time window. The mean is sensitive to outliers, while the median is more robust in the presence of noise or artifacts. These features are widely used in ERP-based paradigms in EEG or ECoG, where stimulus-locked average responses provide crucial information about cognitive processing. However, this technique is generally not very useful for real-time BCI applications, which mostly require single trial-based analysis.
- *Variance and Standard Deviation:* These features quantify the variability or dispersion of the signal. In EEG and ECoG, increased variance can reflect heightened brain activity or noise, while low variance may indicate rest or disengagement. They are simple to compute and often serve as initial features for cognitive state detection in BCI systems.
- *Skewness and Kurtosis:* These higher-order statistical moments measure the asymmetry (skewness) and peakedness or flatness (kurtosis) of the amplitude distribution. Such features can detect abnormal signal distributions, which may occur during seizures intracranial electroencephalography (iEEG) or artifact contamination. These methods are not suitable as features, however, they can enhance ML model performance when combined with other features such as time-domain or spectral.
- *Zero-crossing Rate (ZCR):* ZCR represents the frequency which equates to the number of times a signal crosses the zero amplitude level within a window. It is useful in motor imagery (MI) and sensorimotor tasks for EEG signals, where higher mental effort can modulate this rate. ZCR is also useful for identifying baseline shifts or artifacts.
- *Peak-to-peak Amplitude:* This feature measures the difference between the maximum and minimum values within a time window. It captures the signal's dynamic range and is effective in detecting large deflections, ERP based evoked responses as well as muscle artifacts in EEG and ECoG. It is also used in fNIRS to estimate hemodynamic response amplitudes following stimuli. An example of this technique is the P300 in EEG, where a positive peak is measured around 300 ms poststimulus.
- *Root Mean Square (RMS):* RMS provides a measure of signal power, particularly helpful in distinguishing between active and resting mental states. It is

commonly used in motor execution or imagery tasks in EEG and iEEG and can also track activation levels in fNIRS by capturing amplitude shifts in the hemodynamic signal.

- *Slope and Line Length:* These features quantify the trend or complexity of the signal over time. The slope of a signal segment indicates rising or falling trends in voltage or oxygenation levels depend on modality used, while line length is a complexity measure sensitive to rapid fluctuations. These are particularly useful in seizure detection from iEEG and for capturing cognitive transitions in fNIRS or EEG.
- *Latency and Duration of Events:* For event-related paradigms, the latency to peak or onset, as well as the duration of response windows, can provide information about processing speed or hemodynamic delay. This is especially relevant in ERP analysis from EEG or ECoG and in fNIRS/fMRI to evaluate task-related timing of brain responses.

### 5.3.2 Frequency-domain Features

Frequency-domain features are time-series transformations of the signals into the spectral domain, often through Fast Fourier Transform (FFT), Welch's method, or autoregressive (AR) models. These transformed features capture spectral powers known to be correlated with cognitive processes. Frequency-domain features are very popular in EEG, iEEG, and ECoG-based BCIs, especially of MI tasks which are based on mu, beta, and high gamma bands. Due to the significant dependency on high temporal resolution to produce meaningful information, their application is less common in fNIRS and fMRI, though slow oscillatory trends can still be informative in certain cognitive states. While frequency-domain features are very useful, they need careful windowing and can lose temporal resolution. They are also more computationally demanding than time-domain features and depend on accurate selection of frequency bands.

- *Fast Fourier Transform (FFT):* FFT is one of the most commonly used methods for converting time-domain signals into their frequency components. It decomposes a signal into its constituent sinusoidal components, providing a global view of spectral content. In EEG, ECoG, and iEEG data, FFT is used to compute PSD across bands such as delta, theta, alpha, beta, and gamma, which are associated with attention, motor activity, and cognitive load. While FFT is computationally efficient and straightforward, it assumes signal stationarity and provides no temporal resolution, which may be a limitation in dynamic tasks or short-lived events.
- *Welch's Method:* Welch's method is an improved version of the periodogram approach that reduces spectral variance by dividing the signal into overlapping segments, applying a window function, and averaging the resulting periodograms. This technique is particularly useful for analyzing noisy EEG

or ECoG signals in MI BCIs, where robust spectral estimates are critical. Although it enhances spectral stability, it slightly compromises frequency resolution and assumes the signal is stationary within each windowed segment.

- *Autoregressive (AR) Modeling:* AR modeling fits the signal to a linear combination of its past values, allowing spectral estimation based on model parameters. AR-based methods are advantageous for short data segments and provide smoother spectral estimates than FFT, making them useful in real-time or low-latency applications in EEG and iEEG. AR modelling is also suited for tracking spectral shifts in motor tasks or cognitive transitions. However, it requires model order selection, which can significantly affect accuracy and may be sensitive to noise.
- *Multitaper Spectral Estimation:* The multitaper method applies multiple orthogonal tapers (windowing functions) to the data to obtain a set of independent spectral estimates that are then averaged. This approach improves the bias-variance trade-off in spectral estimation and is particularly useful for short-duration or noisy segments. It has used in high-resolution ECoG and iEEG analysis, especially when examining narrow-band oscillatory activity. While it offers superior spectral concentration and robustness, it is computationally more intensive and requires careful taper selection.
- *Wavelet Transform (Spectral View):* Although wavelets are often classified under time-frequency methods, they can also be used purely for spectral analysis by collapsing the time dimension. Continuous wavelet transform (CWT) provides a multiresolution analysis of frequency content and can detect frequency-specific phenomena such as bursts or oscillatory patterns. In EEG and fNIRS, wavelet-based spectral features are useful for distinguishing mental workload or emotional states. However, the trade-off between time and frequency resolution require a careful management, and interpretation can be less intuitive compared to FFT-based methods.
- *Band Power Features:* Rather than using the full spectrum, band power features are derived by integrating power within predefined frequency bands (e.g., alpha: 8–13 Hz, beta: 13–30 Hz). These are among the most widely used features in BCI, especially for EEG and ECoG MI paradigms. High gamma band power (above 60 Hz) in ECoG and iEEG is often linked to localized cortical activation. Band power features are simple to compute and effective in classification tasks, though their reliability depends on correct band selection and preprocessing.
- *Spectral Entropy:* Spectral entropy measures the disorder or unpredictability in the power spectrum of a signal. It is useful for detecting changes in brain state, such as transitions between rest and task, or levels of consciousness. It has been applied in EEG for workload assessment and in fNIRS to capture cognitive variability. Spectral entropy is very useful, however, it can be sensitive to noise and may not perform well in short or low-SNR recordings.

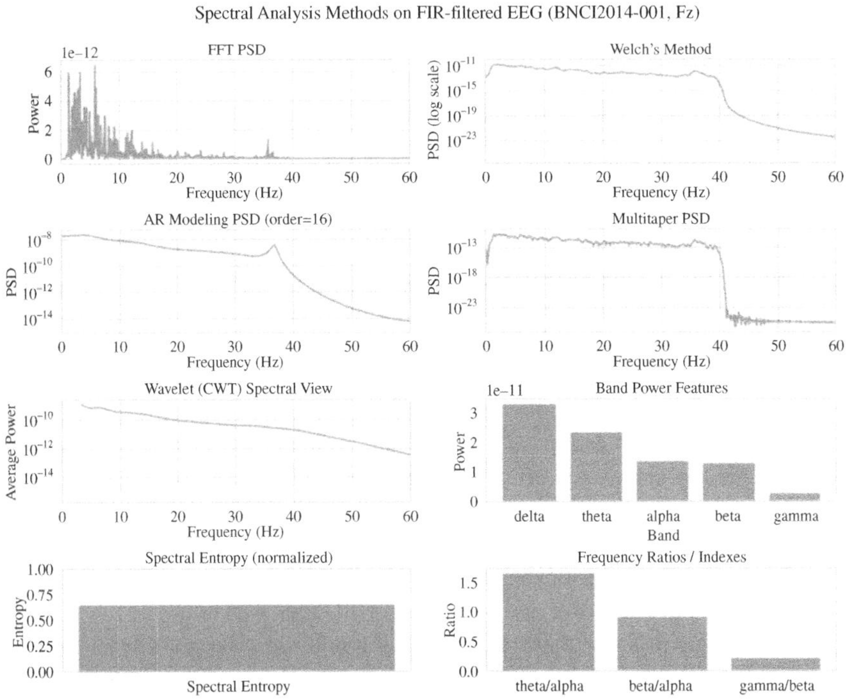


**Figure 5.2** Different frequency domain features applied on raw EEG signals based on BNCI database. *Source*: [64]/Frontiers Media S.A./CC BY 3.0.

- *Frequency Ratios and Indexes:* Ratios of power between different frequency bands (e.g., theta/alpha, beta/alpha) serve as indicators of cognitive or mental state. These features are frequently used in neurofeedback and workload monitoring with EEG and fNIRS. Although simple, they provide interpretable markers for tracking engagement or fatigue. The main limitation lies in their susceptibility to signal artifacts and individual variability.

Figure 5.2 shows an example of EEG signals to extract frequency domain features with different techniques.

### 5.3.3 Time-frequency Features

Time-frequency features aim to capture how frequency content evolves over time, using methods such as the short-time Fourier transform (STFT), Continuous Wavelet Transform (CWT), or Hilbert–Huang transform (HHT). These methods are especially powerful for analyzing nonstationary signals with transient frequency changes, such as task-evoked bursts or cognitive shifts. EEG, ECoG, and iEEG data benefit significantly from time-frequency analysis due to their rapid dynamics and rich spectral content. For fNIRS and fMRI, time-frequency methods are less common but can sometimes help detect periodic vascular responses or hemodynamic delays in block or event-related designs. Time-frequency features offer a detailed view of neural activity but are high-dimensional and computationally intensive. These methods work best in combination of dimensionality reduction or feature selection techniques to avoid overfitting, particularly when data volume is limited.

- *Short-time Fourier Transform (STFT):* STFT involves segmenting the signal into short overlapping windows and applying the Fourier transform to each window. This provides a time-varying spectrum by assuming quasi-stationarity within each segment. STFT is highly interpretable and computationally efficient, making it suitable for real-time applications in EEG and ECoG-based BCIs. However, its fixed time-frequency resolution is a limitation; as a result, short windows generally provide better temporal resolution but poorer frequency resolution, and vice versa. This trade-off makes it less adaptable for capturing rapid changes in frequency, which may occur in iEEG or transient events.
- *Continuous Wavelet Transform (CWT):* CWT decomposes the signal using wavelet functions that vary in scale and shift to offer a multi-resolution time-frequency representation. This technique provides high temporal resolution for high-frequency components and high frequency resolution for low-frequency components. CWT is particularly effective in EEG and ECoG data for detecting transient bursts or rhythms like alpha suppression or gamma activation. The adaptability of CWT also makes it useful for iEEG, where sharp, high-frequency discharges may be relevant (e.g., in epilepsy studies). However, CWT is computationally demanding in comparison to STFT and also require parameter tuning for optimal performance.
- *Hilbert–Huang Transform (HHT):* HHT combines empirical mode decomposition (EMD) with the Hilbert transform, which allows analysis of nonlinear and nonstationary signals. It decomposes a signal into intrinsic mode functions (IMFs) and then computes instantaneous frequency and amplitude. HHT is useful for non-sinusoidal task-related activity commonly found in EEG and ECoG signals. Its high adaptiveness also allows it to capture dynamic spectral changes without the constraints of fixed bases. However, HHT is computationally expensive and less robust in noisy conditions. It has limited application in fNIRS or fMRI due to the slow dynamics and lower signal complexity of those modalities.

- *Multitaper Time-frequency Analysis:* This method enhances spectral estimation by applying multiple orthogonal tapers to reduce variance and spectral leakage. When used in a sliding window fashion, multitaper analysis provides time-frequency representations with improved statistical robustness. It is particularly useful in ECoG and iEEG, where signal quality permits precise spectral measurements. In EEG, it aids in analyzing sustained oscillations during cognitive tasks. Its use in hemodynamic modalities is rare but may be considered for evaluating low-frequency oscillations in resting-state fMRI or task-based fNIRS.
- *Wigner-Ville Distribution (WVD):* WVD is a non-parametric time-frequency analysis method for non-stationary signals like EEGs and iEEG, similar to Fourier transform but offering a two-dimensional map of time-varying frequency characteristics. However, very useful, this method suffers from cross-term interference which may introduce noise in signals in the form of unknown frequencies in the signals. WVD is occasionally applied in EEG and iEEG signals to capture subtle frequency shifts in complex paradigms, such as speech or sound processing. There is limited use of WVD in fNIRS and fMRI due to its sensitivity to slow and overlapping signal components.
- *Stockwell Transform (S-Transform):* S-Transform blends the benefits of STFT and wavelet transforms by providing frequency-dependent resolution while maintaining absolute phase information. This makes it a valuable tool in EEG and ECoG for identifying time-localized phase-locked oscillations. It has also been used in seizure detection and mental workload assessment. However, its computational cost is higher than STFT and CWT, limiting its practicality for large-scale or real-time BCI systems.

Figure 5.3 shows an example of EEG signals to extract time-frequency domain features with different techniques as explained above.

### 5.3.4 Spatial Features

Spatial features utilize the spatial configuration of sensors or reconstructed source activity to extract relevant patterns. Techniques such as CSPs, PCA, ICA, and source localization are used to enhance signal discriminability by isolating task-relevant regions. These methods are particularly effective in multichannel EEG, ECoG, and iEEG recordings, where spatial filtering can emphasize localized neural activity while reducing noise. Spatial features are less prominent in fNIRS and fMRI, though multivariate pattern analysis (MVPA) and region-of-interest (ROI) approaches can still extract spatially informative patterns from these modalities. While spatial filtering enhances SNR and can significantly improve classification accuracy, it often requires a large number of well-defined and

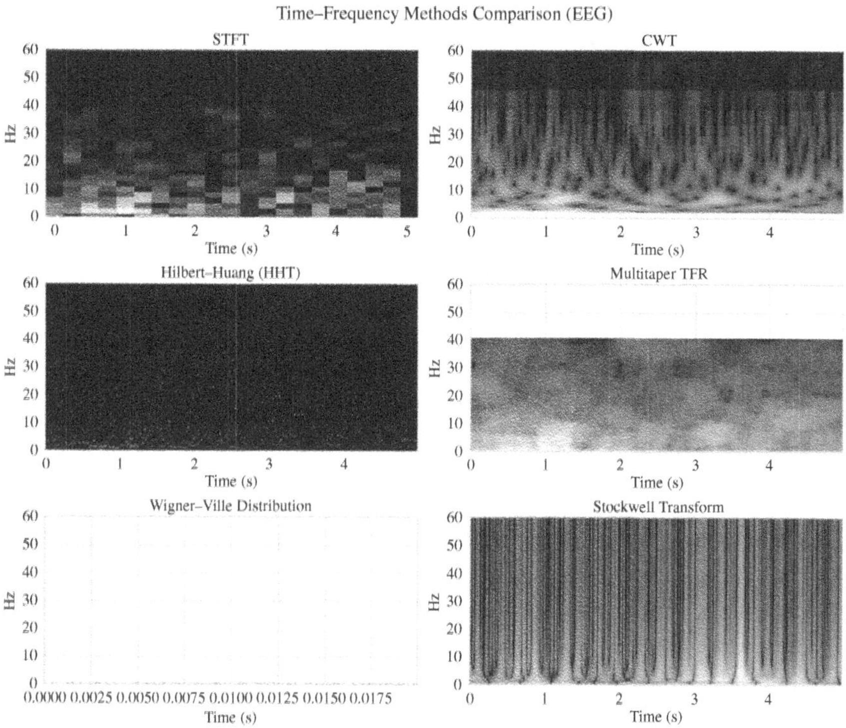


**Figure 5.3** Different time-frequency domain features applied on raw EEG signals based on BNCI database. *Source*: [66]/Frontiers Media S.A./CC BY 3.0.

positioned channels and is sensitive to intersubject variability and head movement. Calibration and data quality play critical roles in the success of these methods.

- *Common Spatial Patterns (CSPs):* CSP is a supervised spatial filtering technique that maximizes the variance difference between two classes (e.g., left vs. right MI) in EEG, ECoG, and iEEG data. It generates spatial filters that project multichannel signals onto components most informative for discrimination. CSP has been widely used for motor imagery-based BCI applications due to its high efficiency and strong performance. However, it requires a sufficient number of trials to produce optimal results. CSP is most commonly used with EEG-based BCIs, and its application in fNIRS is limited.
- *Principal Component Analysis (PCA):* Similar to preprocessing, PCA can also be used to project the data onto orthogonal components that capture the highest variance. It is modality-agnostic and used across EEG, fNIRS, and fMRI

to denoise or compress multichannel or voxel-wise data. PCA is particularly useful for visualization, though it is unsupervised and does not necessarily retain features most relevant to classification tasks. It can serve as a precursor to other spatial filters or ML models.

- *Independent Component Analysis (ICA):* Similar to preprocessing, ICA is also useful to extract spatial features. In EEG and ECoG, ICA can isolate artifacts (e.g., eye blinks, muscle activity) or identify functional sources such as sensorimotor rhythms. In fMRI, ICA is applied in resting-state analysis to identify networks like the default mode network. Although being effective, ICA performance depends on the number of channels and assumptions of statistical independence, and component interpretation may require manual inspection.
- *Source Localization (LORETA and Beamforming):* Source localization techniques attempt to reconstruct the spatial origin of signals recorded at the scalp or cortical surface. These methods aim to solve the inverse problem by estimating the underlying neural sources, often using anatomical constraints from MRI. In EEG and MEG, approaches such as low-resolution electromagnetic tomography (LORETA) or beamforming can reveal task-specific activations. ECoG and iEEG generally has simpled geometry and sensor arrangements, allowing more accurate localization. In fMRI, the signal already reflects spatially localized activity, so direct localization is inherent to the modality. These methods require accurate head models and electrode positions and are computationally intensive.
- *Region-of-Interest (ROI) and Voxel-Based Features:* In fMRI and fNIRS, spatial features are often derived by averaging signals within predefined brain regions or extracting voxel-level statistics. ROI-based features reduce dimensionality and enhance interpretability, especially in task-based or anatomical studies. Voxel-based approaches preserve spatial granularity and are used in ML methods such as support vector machine (SVM) and convolutional neural network (CNN). However, these methods are sensitive to motion artifacts and alignment errors and may require smoothing or normalization steps.
- *Multivariate Pattern Analysis (MVPA):* MVPA involves analyzing spatially distributed patterns of brain activity rather than single-channel responses. It is widely used in fMRI and increasingly applied to EEG and fNIRS to decode cognitive states. By treating spatial patterns as high-dimensional vectors, MVPA can detect subtle differences between experimental conditions, often using classifiers like SVM or logistic regression. MVPA provides strong decoding performance but requires careful cross-validation and suffers from high computational and data demands.
- *Topographical Mapping and Spatial Entropy:* Topographical features involve computing spatial maps of amplitude or power distributions across electrodes. Measures like spatial entropy or center-of-mass can summarize these

maps into compact spatial descriptors. This approach is useful in EEG and ECoG for capturing overall activation patterns during different tasks or mental states. Though less common in fNIRS and fMRI, analogous measures can be derived from cortical surface projections or optical channel grids.

### 5.3.5 Nonlinear and Entropy-based Features

Nonlinear and entropy-based feature extraction techniques aim to provide information about the complexity, irregularity, and chaotic properties of brain signals. Common measures include sample entropy, approximate entropy, fractal dimension, and Lyapunov exponents. These are particularly suited to capturing the dynamical nature of neural activity, which may not be well-represented by linear models. In EEG, ECoG, and iEEG data, these features have been used to detect states of consciousness, attention, or cognitive load. Similarly, entropy-based measures in fMRI and fNIRS can also reflect variability in hamodynamic responses and may correlate with resting-state complexity or pathology. Although nonlinear entropy-based features are robust to noise, they are computationally demanding and highly dependent on parameter settings. They can also be difficult to interpret neurophysiologically and may require domain-specific expertise to apply effectively.

- *Approximate Entropy (ApEn):* ApEn aims to quantify the regularity and unpredictability of fluctuations in a given time-series signals. A lower ApEn indicates more predictable and regular activity, while higher values suggest greater complexity. This method is commonly applied to EEG, ECoG, and iEEG signals for distinguishing cognitive load levels, sleep stages, or seizure events. It has also been used with fNIRS and fMRI to assess the regularity of hemodynamic signals, although the low temporal resolution of these modalities may limit precision.
- *Sample Entropy (SampEn):* SampEn is an improved version of ApEn by avoiding self-matches and providing better consistency for short time-series signals. It is widely used in EEG-based workload monitoring, consciousness assessment, and mental fatigue detection. SampEn has also shown promise in differentiating task-related states in fNIRS and in identifying functional abnormalities in resting-state fMRI data. Compared to ApEn, it is more stable and less dependent on data length, though still sensitive to parameter choices.
- *Multiscale Entropy (MSE):* MSE analyzes the signal at multiple temporal scales, revealing how complexity varies across short and long time horizons. MSE is particularly effective for EEG and iEEG to extract features related to age-related cognitive decline, anesthesia effects, and attention modulation. It can also provide insight into system-level organization and complexity of resting-state activity in fMRI and fNIRS. However, this method is

computationally demanding and significantly depends on preprocessing to ensure meaningful scale interpretation.

- *Fractal Dimension (FD):* FD measures the self-similarity or scaling behavior of a signal. Techniques such as Higuchi's or Katz's method can be used to estimate FD, which has been linked to neural efficiency and cognitive load in EEG and ECoG studies. FD is also applicable in fNIRS to assess brain function during mental tasks and in fMRI for evaluating functional connectivity networks. Although FD offers a compact representation of signal complexity, it is highly sensitive to SNR and filtering technique used.
- *Lyapunov Exponents:* These exponents assess the chaotic nature of a system by measuring divergence of nearby trajectories in phase space. Positive Lyapunov exponents suggest chaos and are used to identify irregular dynamics in seizure detection or sleep transitions using EEG and iEEG. Their application to fNIRS and fMRI is less common due to temporal limitations but remains conceptually viable for slow dynamical systems. The main challenge lies in accurate estimation from noisy or short-duration signals.
- *Lempel–Ziv Complexity (LZC):* LZC quantifies the randomness of a signal by counting distinct patterns in a binary sequence derived from the original signal. It is used in EEG to assess consciousness levels, particularly in clinical settings involving anesthesia or coma. In fMRI, LZC helps characterize resting-state brain dynamics and has been used to differentiate between neurotypical and pathological brain function. This method is relatively robust to noise but requires careful preprocessing for binarization.
- *Permutation Entropy (PE):* PE evaluates the ordinal patterns of the signal rather than raw values, offering robustness to amplitude variations and noise. It has been successfully used in EEG and ECoG for emotion recognition, mental workload classification, and epileptic seizure detection. In fNIRS, PE provides insight into cortical engagement during motor or cognitive tasks. In contrast to several techniques mentioned here, PE is computationally efficient, therefore suitable for real-time BCI applications, though its performance can depend on window size and embedding parameters.

## 5.4 Multimodal Signal Processing Considerations

In multimodal BCI systems (e.g., EEG-fNIRS, EEG-ECoG), preprocessing must be carefully designed to account for differences in sampling rate, signal characteristics, and spatial resolution. A combination of tailored methods is often required:

- *Temporal Synchronization:* Aligns time-series data from different modalities, often with different sampling rates. This step is essential for accurate multimodal integration but requires precise timestamping and synchronization protocols.

- *Spatial Coregistration:* It helps to align sensors and cortical sources across modalities. It also supports spatially informed analyses but requires a complex setup, which includes head models or anatomical imaging data.
- *Cross-modality Normalization:* This normalization is require to adjust for differences in scale and latency between modalities. It may facilitate combining analysis using ML models, although it can oversimplify physiological differences inherent to each signal type.

Effective multimodal signal processing enables robust and informative BCIs by combining complementary strengths of different measurement techniques, e.g., temporal resolution of EEG with spatial or metabolic information from fNIRS or fMRI.

## 5.5 Software Ecosystem for Signal Processing in Brain–Computer Interface (BCIs)

Preprocessing approaches are invaluable for understanding the neural correlates of cognitive functions. However, for effective use in BCIs, especially in real-time applications, these steps must be integrated into automated and reproducible pipeline: Many modern software libraries facilitate this integration. The following ecosystem is organized according to a typical BCI pipeline: classical analysis toolboxes, data acquisition frameworks, automated preprocessing pipelines, modern deep learning tools, and benchmarking or workflow systems.

### 5.5.1 MNE-Python

MNE-Python [68] is a comprehensive open-source Python library for processing MEG, EEG, and fNIRS data. Built with scientific computing in mind, it offers a fully scriptable interface that supports end-to-end workflows, including real-time data acquisition, preprocessing, source localization, and statistical modeling. The library includes implementations for filtering, epoching, event detection, ICAs, and time-frequency analysis.

One of MNE-Python's major advantages is its adherence to the Brain Imaging Data Structure (BIDS) standard, which ensures compatibility and reproducibility in large-scale neuroimaging studies. It also supports interactive visualizations of raw signals, sensor positions, and source estimates. Due to its Python foundation, MNE-Python is highly extensible and easily combined with ML libraries such as scikit-learn and PyTorch, making it a preferred choice for both research and applied BCI development.

### 5.5.2 EEGLAB

EEGLAB [69] is a long-standing MATLAB-based toolbox for EEG analysis, widely used in both academic and clinical research settings. It provides both a graphical user interface (GUI) as well as full scripting capabilities, therefore suitable for all kinds of users with different expertise and knowledge in programming languages. EEGLAB has a vast variety of methods and techniques for data preprocessing, including resampling, filtering, re-referencing, artifact rejection, ICA, and group analysis.

In addition to its core functions, EEGLAB has a modular plugin architecture that allows researchers to integrate community-developed tools for specialized tasks such as source localization, connectivity analysis, or classification. Time-frequency decompositions, ERP image visualization, and statistical comparisons are also well supported. Because of its long-standing development and active user community, EEGLAB remains a staple in EEG-focused BCI pipelines.

### 5.5.3 FieldTrip

FieldTrip [70] is an advanced MATLAB-based toolbox designed for the analysis of electrophysiological data in cognitive neuroscience and clinical research. It supports multiple recording modalities, including EEG, MEG, and ECoG, and offers a highly customizable, script-based environment for processing and analyzing large and complex datasets. Some of key features of FieldTrip include flexible trial definition, advanced artifact rejection methods (manual and automatic), time-frequency analysis, and sophisticated source localization techniques using head models and forward modeling. It is particularly well-suited for studies involving experimental manipulations, source-level EEG/MEG analysis, or multimodal integration. FieldTrip's modular design and emphasis on transparency and reproducibility have contributed to its wide adoption in experimental neuroimaging labs.

### 5.5.4 Lab Streaming Layer

Lab Streaming Layer (LSL) [71] is an open-source software framework designed for the synchronized acquisition and streaming of time-series data such as EEG, EMG, eye-tracking, motion capture, and event markers. LSL provides a network-based interface that allows streaming and collecting physiological data over a network in real-time. One of the key benefits of an LSL-based interface is time synchronization across multiple data streams and automatically compensating for all data latency due to the network. LSL is a popular framework for multimodal and closed-loop BCI systems. This makes it ideal for experimental setups involving several hardware devices, such as simultaneous EEG and eye-tracking, or EEG and TMS. The system architecture allows developers to stream data locally or over networks using platform-independent APIs in C++, Python, MATLAB, Java, and other languages.

LSL is frequently used as a low-latency middleware layer between acquisition hardware and software platforms like MNE-Python and BrainFlow. It supports both data acquisition and event marking, allowing real-time experiments to incorporate user feedback and external experimental events.

### 5.5.5 BrainFlow

BrainFlow [72] is a lightweight, cross-platform software framework designed for real-time data acquisition and preprocessing from a variety of commercial EEG devices. Developed with embedded and mobile BCI applications in mind, BrainFlow provides a unified API for communicating with consumer and research-grade hardware across different operating systems and languages, including Python, C++, Java, and MATLAB. The library includes basic signal processing routines such as filtering, artifact removal, and feature extraction, allowing for rapid prototyping and deployment in resource-constrained environments. Its low-latency architecture and compatibility with wearable hardware make BrainFlow particularly suitable for real-time neurofeedback, closed-loop stimulation, and portable BCI systems. Additionally, BrainFlow can serve as the data acquisition backend for higher-level ML pipelines and interfaces with other libraries such as MNE-Python.

### 5.5.6 PREP Pipeline

The PREP Pipeline (Preprocessing Pipeline) [73] is an automated framework developed for standardized EEG preprocessing in large-scale datasets. It was originally designed to support the analysis of high-density EEG in population-level studies but has broader applicability in any workflow requiring reliable and repeatable preprocessing. The pipeline performs essential steps such as line noise removal, robust average referencing, high-pass filtering, and bad channel interpolation. Its design emphasizes transparency, reproducibility, and minimal manual intervention. PREP is typically implemented in MATLAB and can be used as a preprocessing stage before applying ICA or further statistical modeling in tools like EEGLAB or FieldTrip. By providing standardized outputs, the PREP pipeline facilitates cross-study comparisons and meta-analysis in EEG research.

### 5.5.7 Autoreject

Autoreject [74] is a specialized Python package developed for the automatic detection and repair of bad segments and channels in EEG datasets. Built to integrate seamlessly with MNE-Python, it leverages ML techniques to learn data-driven thresholds for rejecting and interpolating artifact-contaminated trials. Unlike traditional rejection methods that use fixed amplitude or frequency thresholds, Autoreject adapts its behavior to the statistical properties of the data, optimizing both trial-level and channel-level cleaning. It supports cross-validation to select optimal parameters and can operate in both global and local modes, depending on the dataset size and experimental design. By automating the preprocessing pipeline, Autoreject facilitates analysis and improves reproducibility, particularly in large EEG studies or real-time BCI environments.

### 5.5.8 Braindecode

Braindecode [75] is a deep learning toolbox built on top of PyTorch and designed specifically for decoding EEG and ECoG signals. It provides state-of-the-art neural network architectures, including ShallowFBCSPNet, Deep4Net, EEGNet, and hybrid convolutional recurrent models. These architectures are implemented with strong defaults for neural data (e.g., channel-first formats, artifact-aware preprocessing blocks) and can be trained end-to-end on raw or minimally processed data.

A key advantage of Braindecode is its integration with MNE-Python, enabling seamless transitions between classical preprocessing pipelines and deep learning-based approaches. It also provides rich utilities for experiment management, dataset loading, and benchmarking. As ML becomes increasingly central in BCI development, Braindecode serves as one of the main frameworks bridging neuroscience signal processing and modern deep learning.

### 5.5.9 TorchEEG

TorchEEG [76] is also a deep learning library built entirely on PyTorch and designed to support research in EEG-based emotion recognition, cognitive-state decoding, and cross-subject generalization. The library includes over 20 benchmark EEG datasets and provides ready-to-use models for both classification and generative tasks, such as EEGNet, Conv-TasNet variants, graph convolutional networks (GCNs), and transformer-based architectures.

TorchEEG emphasizes data augmentation, self-supervised learning, and generative modeling capabilities that are increasingly important in modern preprocessing workflows. Features such as trial alignment, frequency-band decomposition, and noise synthesis allow researchers to construct advanced pipelines that integrate data cleaning with downstream classification. This makes TorchEEG especially valuable for large-scale or cross-participant BCIs.

### 5.5.10 Deep1010

Deep1010 [77] is a specialized tool for EEG deep learning workflows that provides standardized channel-ordering and spatial embedding schemes based on the international 10–10 and 10–20 systems. Many deep learning models require consistent channel geometry, and Deep1010 ensures compatibility across datasets and acquisition systems. This avoids common pitfalls in cross-dataset generalization, where mismatched channel ordering can degrade performance. Deep1010 is particularly useful when integrating multiple datasets in training deep networks, such as in transfer learning or subject-independent BCI models.

### 5.5.11 NeuroKit2

NeuroKit2 [78] is a Python library designed for comprehensive preprocessing of physiological time-series, including EEG, cardiac, electrodermal, and respiratory signals. It provides modular structure and broad set of signal-cleaning utilities make, which are valuable complements to BCI preprocessing workflows. NeuroKit2 provides high-level functions for filtering, detrending, artifact correction, and event detection and supports multimodal physiological analysis.

NeuroKit2 is frequently used in rapid prototyping, educational contexts, and multimodal BCI pipelines where EEG is accompanied by ECG, EMG, or EDA signals.

### 5.5.12 Mother of All BCI Benchmarks

Mother of All BCI Benchmarks (MOABB) [79] is a Python-based benchmark platform that provides standardized preprocessing and evaluation pipelines for BCI algorithms. It includes dozens of public EEG datasets and ensures fair comparison across algorithms through consistent cross-validation, filtering, and feature-extraction procedures. Although MOABB is primarily designed for algorithm benchmarking rather than real-time preprocessing, it plays a key role in evaluating preprocessing strategies at scale. ML and deep learning models developed using Braindecode or TorchEEG often rely on MOABB for reproducible evaluation.

## 5.6 Relevance to Real-world BCI Applications

Automated signal processing becomes even more crucial when BCIs are deployed outside the laboratory. In uncontrolled environments, users engage in natural behaviors, experience variable emotional and cognitive states, and are influenced by social and environmental context. These factors introduce noise and variability that must be addressed in real time. Automated preprocessing, adaptive feature extraction, and AI-based enhancement allow BCI systems to maintain performance in these complex settings. By combining these techniques into an integrated pipeline, BCI systems can move toward greater robustness, usability, and generalization. The ongoing integration of AI into each stage of signal processing not only improves accuracy but also reduces the burden on users and researchers, paving the way for truly scalable brain-computer interface technologies.

## 5.7 Summary

This chapter has explored the integration of automated signal processing techniques in neural interfaces, particularly BCIs. It outlined how traditional signal processing approaches focused on noise filtering and manual feature extraction have evolved into adaptive, automated pipelines that combine classical methods with automated denoising. Preprocessing steps such as filtering, artifact removal, normalization, and multimodal synchronization were discussed, along with feature extraction techniques in the time, frequency, time-frequency, spatial, and nonlinear domains. Together, these methods provide complementary insights into brain activity and form the basis for robust decoding.

The chapter also highlighted the importance of software ecosystems such as MNE-Python, EEGLAB, FieldTrip, BrainFlow, LSL, Autoreject, and the PREP pipeline in enabling reproducible and scalable workflows. These tools help integrate complex preprocessing and feature extraction steps into end-to-end BCI systems. Building upon this foundation, the next chapter will focus on ML and generative AI methods that operate on these processed signals to perform classification, regression, adaptation, and higher-level neural decoding in real-world applications.

# 6

# Machine Learning and Generative AI for Neural Decoding

Brain signals require critical preprocessing after acquisition, as discussed in Chapter 5; however, interpreting and decoding of these brain signals requires machine learning (ML) techniques. Once the signal is clean, artifacts are removed, and data is transformed into features; ML models can begin taking actions. These actions depend on the context of the dataset and task, such as estimating cognitive states or enabling predictive adaptation. Over the past decade, the ML field has made significant progress, particularly in deep learning (DL), reinforcement learning (RL), transfer learning, and more recently, large-scale generative and foundational models. These methods are well suited for large complex datasets such as neural data, which are generally noisy, temporally structured, and high-dimensional. Alongside broader advances in ML methods, generative and foundation models have opened up new possibilities with neural data, ranging from from prediction to synthetic data generation.

While these advances have transformed the broader field of ML, their impact on neural interfaces is especially significant. This chapter therefore provides a structured overview of learning paradigms and generative approaches as they apply to neural decoding. It first discussed classical and DL methods for neural data analysis, then explores reinforcement and transfer learning for adaptive brain–computer interfaces (BCIs).

## 6.1 ML Methods for Neural Data Analysis

The interpretation and prediction of neural signals in BCI systems rely heavily on ML techniques. This section sheds light on some of the key ML algorithms, including supervised and unsupervised, including deep learning methods.

### 6.1.1 Supervised Learning

Supervised learning is a predictive modeling approach in which the algorithm learns a mapping from inputs to outputs using labeled training data. Formally, given a dataset

$$\mathcal{D} = \{(x_i, y_i)\}_{i=1}^{N},$$

where $x_i \in \mathbb{R}^d$ are input features, $y_i$ are corresponding labels, and $N =$ total number of training samples, the objective is to learn a function $f_\theta : \mathbb{R}^d \rightarrow \mathcal{Y}$ that minimizes an expected loss

$$\min_{\theta} \frac{1}{N} \sum_{i=1}^{N} \mathcal{L}(f_\theta(x_i), y_i) + \lambda\, \Omega(\theta),$$

where $\mathcal{L}$ is a task-specific loss function, for example, cross-entropy is used for classification and mean squared error for regression, $\Omega(\theta)$ is a regularization term and $\lambda$ controls regularization strength.

In the context of BCIs, $x_i$ typically represents feature vectors derived from electroencephalography (EEG), electrocorticography (ECoG), intracranial electroencephalography (iEEG), or functional near-infrared spectroscopy (fNIRS) signals. Common examples include band-power features, functional connectivity metrics, and entropy-based complexity measures. The corresponding labels $y_i$ may encode, for instance, motor imagery (MI) classes such as imagined left vs. right-hand movement, cognitive states such as mental fatigue, attention level, mental workload, discrete command sets, or continuous control variables such as cursor position.

#### 6.1.1.1 Most Commonly Used Supervised ML Models

Several models are commonly used and popular in supervised learning for neural decoding:

- **Linear discriminant analysis (LDA):** LDA aims to project data onto a low-dimensional subspace and use it to separate classes by maximizing and minimizing variance between classes and within classes, respectively. LDA seeks a projection $w$ maximizing

$$J(w) = \frac{w^\top \Sigma_B w}{w^\top \Sigma_W w},$$

  where $J(w)$ is the Fisher discriminant criterion, $w$ is the projection vector, $\sum_B$ is the between-class covariance matrix, $\sum_w$ is the within-class covariance matrix. LDA is widely used in MI BCIs due to its simplicity, robustness, and good performance on small datasets. There are several LDA variants which have been developed to address common challenges in neural data, including high dimensionality and limited samples. These include Regularized LDA (using shrinkage to stabilize covariance estimates), Stepwise LDA (popular in P300-based BCIs for joint feature selection and classification), Bayesian LDA (incorporating priors to improve generalization), Heteroscedastic LDA (relaxing the equal-covariance assumption), Kernel LDA (for nonlinear class boundaries), and Local Fisher Discriminant Analysis (which preserves local structure in high-dimensional EEG spaces).

- **Support vector machines (SVMs):** SVMs find a hyperplane that maximally separates classes using margin-based optimization. In the linear case, the classifier solves

$$\min_{w,b} \frac{1}{2}\|w\|^2 + C\sum_{i=1}^{N} \xi_i \quad \text{s.t. } y_i(w^\top x_i + b) \geq 1 - \xi_i, \xi_i \geq 0,$$

where $w$ is the normal vector defining the separating hyperplane, $b$ is the bias or intercept term, $\xi_i$ is the slack variable for sample $i$, $C$ is a penalty parameter controlling the trade-off between margin maximization and classification error, $x_i$ is input vector, $y_i$ is the corresponding class label. SVMs are widely used in BCI because they are robust to high-dimensional, low sample size, which is quite common in EEG and ECoG recordings. Several SVM variants are used in neural decoding: linear SVMs for efficient classification with CSP features; kernel SVMs (e.g., RBF, polynomial) for modeling nonlinear neural patterns; least-squares SVMs (LS-SVMs) for fast training suitable for online BCIs; one-class SVMs for novelty detection or unsupervised labeling; and incremental SVMs for adapting to nonstationarity during prolonged sessions. Multi-class schemes such as one-vs-one and one-vs-rest allow SVMs to scale to multi-command BCIs. This versatility and strong generalization ability make SVMs a standard choice in many competition, such as BCI Competition III [80] and IV [64], where they consistently achieved top performance in MI and ERP/P300 decoding tasks.

- **Logistic regression:** Logistic regression is a probabilistic linear classifier modeling

$$p(y = 1|x) = \sigma(w^\top x + b),$$

where $p(y = 1|x)$ is the probability that input $x$ belongs to class 1, $\sigma(\cdot)$ is the logistic sigmoid function, $w$ is the weight vector, $b$ is the bias term and $x$ is the input feature vector. Although logistic regression is a linear classifier, it still performs well with small datasets and is popular in BCI experiments where calibration sessions are short. Its probabilistic outputs allow for well calibrated confidence scores useful in adaptive and RL-based BCIs. Variants such as $\ell_1$-regularized logistic regression enable sparse feature selection by selecting informative EEG channels, while $\ell_2$-regularization improves stability in noisy settings. Multinomial logistic regression supports multi-class decoding tasks, and Bayesian logistic regression provides uncertainty estimates particularly useful when controlling safety critical assistive devices. Due to its interpretability and efficiency, logistic regression is often used as a baseline or as a final classifier in CSP- or PCA-based pipelines.

- **Decision trees and random forests:** Decision trees aim to recursively partition the feature space by axis-aligned splits. These splits are optimized for information gain and Gini impurity-related criteria. Such a participation provides interpretable decision rules and, more importantly, captures nonlinear interactions. This property is very attractive for heterogeneous neural features such as combinations of time-frequency features, entropy, and connectivity features but is also prone to overfitting data. On the other hand, random forests offer a solution to overfitting limitations. They use an ensemble of trees on bootstrapped data with random feature sets for training. This property of random forests improves robustness, reduces variance, and makes them feasible for data with complex and non-linear relationships, often the case of neural signals. In BCIs, random forests are majorly used for event-related potentials (ERPs), mental state estimation, as well as hybrid BCIs combining EEG with physiological sensors such as EEG-EMG and EEG-fNIRS. There are also other variants of these methods such as extremely randomized trees (ExtraTrees) and gradient boosted trees (XGBoost and LightGBM). These trees can allow increased randomness to improve generalization and large-scale offline decoding tasks. All of these methods offer effective BCI prediction and estimation performance with low computation requirements.
- **Multilayer perceptrons (MLPs):** MLPs are feedforward neural networks composed of one or more hidden layers with nonlinear activations (ReLU, tanh, GELU). As universal function approximators, they can learn arbitrarily complex mappings from handcrafted features or even from small windows of raw neural signals. MLPs have been applied to motor imagery (MI) decoding, ERP classification, mental state detection, and hybrid BCI tasks. Variants commonly used in BCI include deep MLPs with multiple hidden layers; sparse MLPs with $\ell_1$ constraints to automatically select relevant neural features; and dropout regularized MLPs to prevent overfitting in small datasets. MLP methods are very effective in combination with feature extraction techniques and while keeping low computational requirements. Although deep learning variants of MLP such as convolutional neural networks (CNNs) and recurrent neural networks (RNNs) perform well if enough neural data is available, MLP still can offer fast inference and low latency for BCI applications.

- **Fuzzy logic and neuro-fuzzy networks:** Fuzzy logic is a computational framework in which variables can take on continuous degrees of truth rather than binary true/false values. This allows fuzzy models to provide soft decision boundaries that are well suited to the uncertainty and nonstationarity inherent in electroencephalography (EEG) and electrocorticography (ECoG) data. Adaptive neuro-fuzzy inference systems (ANFIS), fuzzy C-means clustering, and type-2 fuzzy logic classifiers have been applied to MI, ERP detection, and mental-state decoding. Fuzzy models work well with noisy and low-data regimes and learn interpretable rule-based decisions. This combination is well suited for real-world BCI applications.
- **Riemannian geometry classifiers:** Riemannian geometry methods are based on distance and average defined along geodesics in curved space where standard Euclidean operations do not work. This approach aligns naturally with the structure of EEG covariance matrices. Methods such as minimum distance to Riemannian mean (MDRM) and tangent-space mapping classify trials based on geodesic distances, yielding state-of-the-art performance in MI BCIs. Riemannian approaches avoid distortions introduced by Euclidean operations on covariance matrices and provide exceptional robustness to noise, session variability, and subject-specific differences.
- **Graph-based and graph neural network (GNN) approaches:** Neural data represent spatial and temporal information alongside functional connectivity patterns. This property can be represented by a graph, which is the basis of graph-based models. These models use sensors in EEG or ECoG, as a node and the relation between these sensors, such as proximity, anatomical structure, or functionality, as an edge. Classical graph-learning approaches include methods based on graph Laplacians, spectral graph filtering, and graph-regularized dimensionality reduction, which encourage smoothness of neural features over the graph structure.

  More recently, GNNs have emerged as powerful models for decoding neural activity by learning from both node-level features and network topology. There are several variants of graph models based on convolutional networks, attention networks, spatial-temporal and dynamic graph networks. These variants have been applied in BCI tasks such as MI, mental state and emotion prediction for affective computing, and seizure detection. Graph-based models are very good at handling non-stationarity in neural data by capturing spatial relationships such as sensor dependencies and adaptation to subject-specific features while incorporating time-varying graph structures. Additionally, graph-based models are known to work well with multimodal BCIs as well as by forming subgraphs within a large heterogeneous graph.

#### 6.1.1.2 Evaluation Metrics for BCIs

It is often straightforward to train an ML model, but determining which model is most appropriate can be challenging, especially in BCIs where performance varies across subjects, sessions, and experimental conditions. This makes a clear understanding of performance metrics essential. Effective evaluation requires both the use of appropriate loss functions during training and the selection of meaningful metrics during validation to reflect real-world BCI performance. In classification-based BCIs, two loss functions are used particularly often:

- *Cross-entropy loss:* Used in probabilistic and DL-based models, especially for multi-class problems with softmax outputs, including logistic regression, naïve Bayes variants, deep feedforward networks, CNNs, RNNs/Long Short-Term Memory (LSTM), transformers, and Bayesian neural networks.

$$\mathcal{L} = -\sum_{i=1}^{N} \log p_\theta(y_i \mid x_i).$$

  where $\mathcal{L}$ is the total cross-entropy loss over the dataset, N is the number of samples, $x_i$ is the input sample, $y_i$ is its true class label, and $p(y_i \mid x_i)$ is the predicted probability.
- *Hinge loss:* Employed in margin-based classifiers such as SVMs and its variant,

$$\mathcal{L} = \sum_{i=1}^{N} \max\left(0,\ 1 - y_i(w^\top x_i)\right).$$

  where $\mathcal{L}$ is the total hinge loss, $N$ is the number of training samples, $x_i$ is the input vector, $y_i \in \{-1, +1\}$ is the true binary label, $w$ is the model weight vector, and $w^\top x_i$ is the classifier score.

Once trained, models are assessed using performance metrics that reflect both accuracy and usability in real-world BCI scenarios. Following evaluation measures should be included:

- **Accuracy** and **balanced accuracy**. Let TP, TN, FP, and FN denote the number of true positives, true negatives, false positives, and false negatives, respectively. The overall accuracy is defined as

$$\mathrm{Acc} = \frac{\mathrm{TP} + \mathrm{TN}}{\mathrm{TP} + \mathrm{TN} + \mathrm{FP} + \mathrm{FN}}.$$

  For multi class problems with $K$ classes, let $\mathrm{TP}_k$ and $\mathrm{FN}_k$ denote the true positives and false negatives for class $k$. The recall of class $k$ is

$$\mathrm{Rec}_k = \frac{\mathrm{TP}_k}{\mathrm{TP}_k + \mathrm{FN}_k},$$

and the balanced accuracy is the average recall across classes

$$\text{BAcc} = \frac{1}{K}\sum_{k=1}^{K} \text{Rec}_k.$$

Balanced accuracy is especially important when classes are imbalanced, such as in event-related potential (ERP) detection tasks where target events are rare.

- **Area under the ROC curve (AUC)**. AUC is a measure to evaluate a binary classifier that generates a continuous score $s(x)$, based on the receiver operating characteristic (ROC) curve, which plots the true positive rate against the false positive rate as the decision threshold varies. In the continuous limit, the AUC can be written as:

$$\text{AUC} = \int_0^1 \text{TPR}(\text{FPR})\, d\, \text{FPR},$$

where TPR is the true positive rate and FPR is the false positive rate. In practice, the integral is approximated from a finite set of thresholds by numerical integration, for example, by the trapezoidal rule. AUC is threshold independent and is particularly useful for binary or one versus rest decoding tasks.

- **Information transfer rate (ITR)**. ITR quantifies the effective communication rate of a BCI in bits per unit time by combining classification accuracy and selection speed. For a system with $M$ possible commands and selection accuracy $P$, the information per selection in bits is:

$$I = \log_2 M + P\log_2 P + (1-P)\log_2\left(\frac{1-P}{M-1}\right).$$

If each selection requires $T$ seconds on average, the ITR in bits per minute is

$$\text{ITR} = \frac{60}{T} I.$$

This measure is central in practical BCI evaluation because it reflects both reliability and speed of communication.

- **Confusion matrices**. For a $K$ class problem, the confusion matrix $C \in \mathbb{N}^{K\times K}$ contains entries:

$$C_{ij} = \text{number of samples with true class } i \text{ predicted as class } j.$$

Row $i$ summarizes the prediction distribution for true class $i$, and column $j$ summarizes all samples predicted as class $j$. From $C$ one can derive class specific recalls:

$$\text{Rec}_i = \frac{C_{ii}}{\sum_{j=1}^{K} C_{ij}}$$

and precisions:

$$\text{Prec}_j = \frac{C_{jj}}{\sum_{i=1}^{K} C_{ij}},$$

which provide detailed insight into systematic error patterns and class-specific performance.

Reliable performance assessment also depends on appropriate validation strategies. Cross validation (CV) methods such as k-fold or nested CV are used to obtain unbiased performance estimates and tune hyperparameters. In BCI research, however, it is particularly important that data splits reflect the intended deployment scenario, for example, using trial-wise, session-wise, or subject-wise partitions to avoid overly optimistic estimates and to ensure realistic generalization to new sessions or users.

#### 6.1.1.3 Practical Considerations in Supervised Learning-based BCIs

Supervised learning in BCIs faces several recurring challenges:

- *Limited labeled data:* Recording sessions are time-consuming and tiring for users, so datasets tend to be small. This increases the risk of overfitting, favoring simpler models or strong regularization.
- *Nonstationarity:* Neural signals are known to drift over time due to various factors such as fatigue, artifacts or even disturbances in electrode positions. Therefore, a model trained on earlier data may not work on drifted data anymore.
- *Inter-subject variability:* Neural signatures between participants could overlap but also vary significantly, therefore limiting models' ability to work across participants. Such issues motivate methods like transfer learning (Section 6.1.5).
- *Real-time constraints:* BCI applications need to work in real-time with low latency therefore a model must perform within these constraints.

### 6.1.2 Unsupervised Learning

In contrast to supervised approaches, *unsupervised learning* seeks to learn hidden structure or intrinsic patterns within data that lack explicit labels. Given a dataset $X = \{x_1, x_2, \dots, x_N\}$ with no associated targets, the objective is to model the underlying data distribution, identify natural groupings, or derive compact representations through dimensionality reduction. Unsupervised learning is very useful for exploratory data analysis, including feature discovery, artifacts detection, and extracting the latent brain states. Such outputs are useful for BCIs, especially to understand the data and extract features. In fact, unsupervised learning is often a predecessor step for supervised learning and provides a cleaner, informative, and interpretable representation of neural data. Let's look at some of commonly known unsupervised methods:

#### 6.1.2.1 Clustering Methods

- **K-Means clustering:** K-means partitions data into $k$ clusters by minimizing the within-cluster sum of squared distances:

$$\min_{\{C_k\}} \sum_{j=1}^{k} \sum_{x_i \in C_k} \|x_i - \mu_k\|^2,$$

  where $k$ is the number of clusters, $C_k$ is the set of samples assigned to cluster, $\mu_k$ is the centroid of cluster. In neural signal analysis, k-means can be used to segment recurring brain states, identify resting-state patterns, or group trials with similar temporal or spectral characteristics. Several variants have been applied in BCI settings, including *k-means++* for improved initialization, *kernel k-means* for clustering data with nonlinear relationships which is very useful for time-frequency or connectivity features, and *online k-means* for adapting to nonstationary EEG streams during real-time use.
- **Gaussian mixture models (GMMs):** GMMs represent the data distribution as a mixture of $k$ Gaussian components,

$$p(x) = \sum_{j=1}^{k} \pi_k \mathcal{N}(x \mid \mu_k, \Sigma_k),$$

  $p(x)$ is the probability density, $k$ is the number of Gaussian mixture components, $\pi_k$ is the mixture weight of component, $\mathcal{N}(x \mid \mu_k, \Sigma_k)$ denotes the Gaussian density with mean $\mu_k$ and covariance matrix $\Sigma_k$. Unlike k-means, GMMs assign data points probabilistically (soft clustering) and allow clusters with full covariance structures, making them more flexible for neural data that often exhibit anisotropic or elongated shapes in feature space. Specific variants of GMM relevant to BCIs are diagonal-covariance GMMs that allow representation of high-dimensional features, and Bayesian GMMs that allow extraction of number of mixture components from data. The Hidden Markov model (HMM) can extend the GMM through hidden states and transition probabilities of a sequence of observations. This approach is useful for identifying sequential mental states or tasks in BCI data.
- **Spectral clustering:** Spectral clustering uses the eigenvectors of a similarity (affinity) matrix derived from pairwise distances to embed data into a low-dimensional spectral space, where conventional clustering such as k-means is applied. This enables the discovery of complex, nonlinearly separable structures that are common in neural patterns. In BCIs, spectral clustering has been applied to cluster connectivity matrices, identify functional brain networks, and group trials with similar time-frequency signatures.

There are several variants of spectral clustering, which include normalized and multi-view clustering, specially applicable for multimodal data such as EEG-fNIRS. Other variants include spectral embedding with kernelized affinity functions-based clustering, which allows learning higher-order relationships in neural data.

#### 6.1.2.2 Dimensionality Reduction and Representation Learning

- **Principal component analysis (PCA):** PCA allows projecting data onto orthogonal axes for maximal variance. As discussed in Chapter 5, this method is very useful for dimensional reductions by arranging information based on dominating features specially when dealing with multichannel modality such as EEG, ECoG, and fNIRS data.
- **Independent component analysis (ICA):** Although often discussed as a preprocessing tool for artifact removal, ICA is fundamentally an unsupervised method that decomposes multivariate data into statistically independent components. Beyond artifact removal as discussed in Chapter 5, ICA can reveal latent functional sources and networks.
- **Nonlinear embeddings (t-SNE/UMAP):** t-distributed Stochastic Neighbor Embedding (t-SNE) and Uniform Manifold Approximation and Projection (UMAP) provide low-dimensional embeddings that preserve local neighborhood structure. They are particularly useful to visualize class structure or subject-specific clusters in high-dimensional feature spaces and to detect outliers or rare neural states.
- **Autoencoders:** Neural network-based dimensionality reduction models consisting of an encoder $h = f_\phi(x)$ and decoder $\hat{x} = g_\psi(h)$, trained to minimize reconstruction error. Latent codes $h$ can serve as compact representations for downstream supervised tasks or for clustering.

#### 6.1.2.3 Other Less Common Unsupervised Methods

- **Self-organizing maps (SOMs):** SOMs are competitive learning neural algorithms that project high-dimensional data onto a low-dimensional grid while preserving topological relationships. By organizing inputs according to similarity, SOMs facilitate visualization of EEG feature spaces, clustering of subject-specific neural patterns, and detection of transitions between cognitive states. They have been used in vigilance studies, ERP analysis, and microstate segmentation.
- **Expectation–Maximization (EM) framework:** EM is a general iterative method for maximum-likelihood estimation in models with latent variables. It alternates between estimating hidden variables (E-step) and updating model parameters (M-step). Many unsupervised models used in BCIs, including GMMs and HMM, are special cases of EM. Artifacts, latent

brain states, and mixture-based spectral patterns can all be inferred within the EM framework.

- **Affinity propagation:** This method identifies clusters by passing real-valued messages between data points to determine exemplar samples that best represent each cluster. Unlike k-means, it does not require specifying the number of clusters a priori. Affinity propagation has been applied to cluster EEG microstates, connectivity patterns, and spectral signatures, offering flexibility when cluster structure is unknown or irregular.
- **Fuzzy C-means (FCM) clustering:** FCM generalizes k-means by allowing each data point to belong to multiple clusters with varying degrees of membership. The optimization objective is

$$J = \sum_{i=1}^{N}\sum_{k=1}^{k} u_{ik}^{m} \|x_i - \mu_k\|^2,$$

where $N$ is the number of data points, $k$ is the number of clusters, $u_{ik}$ is the membership degree of data point in cluster $k$, $m > 1$ is the fuzziness parameter controlling the softness of cluster assignments, $x_i$ data, and $\mu_k$ is the centroid of cluster. FCM is particularly effective for noisy EEG data and has been used for artifact detection, mental-state segmentation, and clustering of time–frequency representations.
- **Independent subspace analysis (ISA):** ISA extends ICA by identifying groups of statistically independent subspaces rather than fully independent components. This allows capturing structured dependencies among neural sources, such as coordinated sensorimotor rhythms or frontal midline theta networks. ISA provides a richer decomposition of EEG and ECoG signals than ICA when components naturally cluster into functional modules.

### 6.1.3 Deep Learning

DL refers to a class of ML models composed of multiple layers of nonlinear transformations, capable of learning hierarchical representations directly from raw or minimally processed input data. Over the past decade, DL has advanced rapidly across virtually all areas of ML, including neural interfaces. DL became very popular due to its ability to capture features from temporal, spatial, as well as multimodal relationships in a single model and is extensively utilized in complex brain signals such as EEG, ECoG, iEEG, fNIRS, and fMRI. Let's look at some of most commonly used DL models in neural interfaces:

#### 6.1.3.1 Convolutional Neural Networks

CNNs apply localized filtering and weight sharing to extract spatial, temporal, and spatiotemporal patterns in neural signals. They are especially effective for EEG,

ECoG, and iEEG due to their ability to learn structured features without requiring handcrafted features or feature extractors such as CSP or spectral bands. Common architectural variants include:

- *1D temporal convolutions:* Filters slide along the time axis for each channel, capturing temporal structures such as oscillations, transient bursts, or event-related potentials.
- *2D channel–time convolutions:* Neural data arranged as a channel-by-time matrix allow CNNs to learn joint spatiotemporal patterns, including coordinated cortical activation or propagating waves.
- *Topographic convolutions:* Electrodes mapped onto a 2D grid reflecting scalp geometry enable CNNs originally designed for images to exploit spatial locality and neuroanatomical structure.
- *Frequency-aware CNNs:* Transforming inputs into time–frequency maps such as spectrograms, scalograms that allows CNNs to model spectral dynamics alongside temporal evolution.

Pooling operations (max or average) reduce dimensionality and introduce invariance, while deeper convolutional layers capture increasingly abstract neural features. Batch normalization, dropout, and weight decay are commonly used to stabilize training and prevent overfitting.

#### 6.1.3.2 Recurrent and Sequence Models

Recurrent and sequence-based models capture temporal dependencies in neural time series, making them suitable for continuous decoding and cognitive-state tracking. Basic RNNs maintain a hidden state evolving over time:

$$h_t = \phi(W_h h_{t-1} + W_x x_t + b),$$

where $h_t$ and $x_t$ is the hidden state and input data at time step $t$, $W_h$ is the recurrent weight matrix, $W_x$ is the input weight matrix, $b$ is the bias vector, and $\phi(\cdot)$ is a nonlinear activation function such as tanh or ReLU. While RNNs can express rich sequential dynamics, they often suffer from vanishing and exploding gradients.

RNN has several advanced variants as follows:

- **Long short-term memory (LSTM) and gated recurrent units (GRU):** These are RNN architectures that capture temporal sequences by using gating mechanisms that regulate information flow and preserve long-term dependencies. Such mechanisms address gradient instabilities, and LSTMs and GRUs are widely used in BCIs for decoding continuous trajectories, modeling long-range dependencies, and tracking cognitive processes.
- **Temporal convolutional networks (TCNs):** TCNs employ multiple layers of causal convolutions with large receptive fields, providing stable gradients and efficient parallelization. They offer strong performance for modeling long-duration neural activity and continuous control tasks.

- **Hybrid CNN–RNN architectures:** Convolutional layers extract spatial or spectral features that are then processed by recurrent layers, yielding effective models for MI decoding, speech-related neural signals, or multimodal integration.

These sequential models can operate directly on raw time series or on sequences of derived features such as, band power, entropy, and connectivity computed over sliding windows. They support both discrete classification and continuous prediction.

#### 6.1.3.3 Attention Mechanisms and Transformers

Attention mechanisms compute pairwise interactions between elements in a sequence, enabling a model to selectively focus on salient time points, channels, or spatial regions. Transformer architectures, built from stacked self-attention blocks and feedforward layers, have recently emerged as powerful methods for neural decoding due to their ability to model long-range dependencies without recurrence or convolution. Key transformer variants used in BCIs include:

- *Temporal transformers:* These transformers treat temporal information as tokens and learn their dependencies across long windows without relying on recurrent connections.
- *Spatiotemporal transformers:* In addition to using temporal information, these transformers also consider sensor-time pairs as tokens, enabling flexible modeling of interactions across space and time.
- *Multimodal transformers:* They process neural signals and additionally modalities such as audio, vision, or text jointly, enabling applications such as brain-to-text or brain-to-image generation possible.

Transformers generally require larger datasets and careful regularization, but they offer high modeling capacity and a natural interface with modern foundation models in language and vision.

#### 6.1.3.4 Training, Regularization, and Interpretability

Training deep neural models for BCIs involves significant effort toward parameter optimization and robust regularization due to the small datasets and nonstationary nature of neural recordings:

- *Optimization:* Stochastic gradient descent and variants such as Adam or Root Mean Square Propagation (RMSProp) are commonly used, often combined with learning-rate schedules, gradient clipping, and early stopping to ensure stable convergence.
- *Regularization:* Techniques including dropout, weight decay, batch normalization, and data augmentation like channel dropout, temporal jittering, and

mixup-like feature blending help improve generalization and mitigate overfitting.

- There are several techniques for interpretation; however, some of the commonly used are saliency maps, class activation maps, layer-wise relevance propagation, and occlusion analysis. These techniques aim to provide information about feature relevance with spatial information, dominance of temporal segments, and frequency bands. Such approaches are very important for enhancing trust and transparency in the models.

### 6.1.4 Reinforcement Learning

RL aims to make decisions through trial and error to maximize a numerical reward for an agent that interacts with an environment in a sequential decision-making process. In BCIs, RL is particularly suited for adaptive systems personalization, adjust difficulty, or tune parameters based on performance and feedback.

#### 6.1.4.1 Formalization and Algorithms

RL can be described as a Markov decision process (MDP), defined by $(\mathcal{S}, \mathcal{A}, \mathcal{P}, \mathcal{R}, \gamma)$. The agent's goal is to maximize:

$$J(\pi) = \mathbb{E}\left[\sum_{t=0}^{\infty} \gamma^t r_t \mid \pi\right].$$

$J(\pi)$ is the expected cumulative discounted return under policy $\pi$, $\mathbb{E}_\pi[\cdot]$ denotes expectation when actions are chosen according to policy $\pi$, $\gamma \in [0, 1]$ is the discount factor, $r_t$ is the reward received, and $s_0$ is the initial state.

Key algorithmic families include:

- **Value-based methods include Q-Learning, Deep Q-Networks:** Learn an action-value function $Q(s, a)$ and derive a policy by acting greedily with respect to $Q$ value of that action at that state.
- **Policy gradient methods:** Parameterize a stochastic policy $\pi_\theta(a|s)$ and optimize $J(\theta)$ using gradient ascent:

$$\nabla_\theta J(\theta) \approx \mathbb{E}[\nabla_\theta \log \pi_\theta(a|s)\, R],$$

  where $R$ is a return estimate and $E[\cdot]$ denotes expectation.
- **Actor–critic methods:** Combine an actor (policy) and a critic (value function), often improving stability and data efficiency.
- **Bandit algorithms:** If there are no state dynamics known, such as stimulus selection, bandit algorithms can be used to select actions that can maximize the expected rewards.

#### 6.1.4.2 Applications in BCIs

Some of well known RL applications in BCIs include:

- *Adaptive classifier tuning:* Adjusting decision thresholds, class priors, or feature weights based on ongoing performance feedback.
- *Stimulus selection and adaptive paradigms:* Choosing which stimuli to present, for example, letters to flash in a P300 speller to maximize information gain or user comfort.
- *Control policies for prosthetics and robotics:* Learning mappings from decoded intent or high-level commands to low-level actuator commands, possibly in combination with model-based control strategies.
- *User state-aware adaptation:* Modifying task difficulty, feedback intensity, or interaction modality based on inferred user fatigue, workload, or emotional state.

RL-based applications are driven by reward functions. and these functions could derive rewards from user ratings, task performance like reaction time, physiological markers, as well as brain signals such as error-related potentials, attention, etc.

### 6.1.5 Transfer Learning

As we discussed before, non-stationarity of signals is the key issue with neural data, where it faces inter-subject variability, session-to-session performance change, and limited labeling. The transfer learning aims to address this challenge by training a model on the subject, session, or task to improve performance on a related target domain, subject, session, or task.

Let $\mathcal{D}_S = \{(x_i^S, y_i^S)\}$ and $\mathcal{D}_T = \{(x_j^T, y_j^T)\}$ be the source and target domains, with possibly different distributions $P_S(X, Y)$ and $P_T(X, Y)$. Transfer learning aims to leverage knowledge from $\mathcal{D}_S$ to improve performance on $\mathcal{D}_T$.

#### 6.1.5.1 Fine-tuning and Parameter Sharing

A common approach is to pre-train a model on $\mathcal{D}_S$ and then fine-tune it on $\mathcal{D}_T$:

- Freeze early layers (which capture generic features) and update only later layers task or user specific.
- Use a smaller learning rate for pre-trained layers and a larger one for new layers.
- Optionally, gradually unfreeze layers as more target data become available.

Fine-tuning is particularly effective when architectures are deep and source data are large and diverse in a case like multi-subject datasets.

#### 6.1.5.2 Domain Adaptation

Domain adaptation explicitly reduces the discrepancy between source and target distributions:

- *Feature alignment:* It aims to minimize as maximum mean discrepancy (MMD) between source and target feature distributions in a shared latent space.
- *Adversarial domain adaptation:* It introduces a domain discriminator network trained to distinguish source from target features, while the feature extractor is trained to fool it, encouraging domain-invariant features.
- *Subspace alignment and covariance matching:* It aims to align principal component subspaces or covariance structures across subjects or sessions.

These techniques can be combined with supervised targets when some labels in $\mathcal{D}_T$ are available or used in semi-supervised/unsupervised adaptation.

#### 6.1.5.3 Multi-task Learning

Multi-task learning (MTL) trains a single model to perform several related tasks simultaneously, allowing shared representations to be learned across tasks, conditions, or subjects. By exploiting common structure in neural activity, MTL can improve data efficiency, enhance generalization, and reduce overfitting properties. In MTL frameworks, lower layers typically learn shared features, which include features like temporal filters, spatial patterns, and spectral representations, while task-specific layers provide specialized outputs for each prediction target. Examples of MTL strategies in neural interface include:

- *Joint decoding of multiple cognitive or MI:* A single model that can predict multiple BCI phenomena such as MI, mental states, and intention from the same neural data such as EEG. Such model shares the same learning layer to capture general neural dynamics while following specific layers to learn specific task-specific features.
- *Cross-subject learning with personalized output layers:* A shared backbone is trained on multiple subjects, while each subject has its own output head to account for individual variability. This reduces calibration time and improves transferability across users.
- *Learning shared features across modalities or sensor types:* For multimodal BCIs (EEG–fNIRS, EEG–EMG), MTL can jointly learn modality specific decoders while sharing common spatio-temporal representations across modalities.
- *Combining discrete and continuous outputs:* A single model architecture can classify discrete mental states, left vs. right MI while also regressing continuous control variables like cursor trajectories.

- *Auxiliary-task learning:* Adding auxiliary tasks such as predicting spectral band power, artifact probability, or electrode quality, can regularize the model and guide it toward physiologically meaningful representations. Even if auxiliary labels are weak or noisy, they often can improve the main task.
- *Domain adaptation using task-specific heads:* In settings involving large domain shifts due to different sessions, electrode montages, recording devices, etc. MTL can align shared features while allowing domain specific heads to adapt outputs to each distribution.

MTL frameworks can be implemented using various architectures, including shared CNN backbones, transformer encoders with multiple prediction heads, or recurrent models with branching output layers. By leveraging shared structure across tasks or users, MTL can improve robustness and flexibility, making it a powerful approach for developing generalized and user-adaptive BCIs.

## 6.2 Applications of Generative AI in Neural Interfaces

Generative AI including foundational models is emerging as one of the most influential and rapidly growing fields, with applications in almost every area of science, including neural interfaces. Generative models offer novel capabilities for simulation, augmentation, and brain-driven generation. By leveraging advanced models such as generative adversarial networks (GANs), variational autoencoders (VAEs), diffusion models, and multimodal transformer architectures, researchers are now able to push beyond traditional decoding paradigms toward more creative, adaptive, and human-aligned interactions.

Table 6.1 summarizes several key areas where generative AI is making impactful contributions to neural interface technologies.

### 6.2.1 Synthetic Neural Data Generation with Generative Models

One of the foundational applications of generative AI in neural interfaces is the creation of synthetic neural data. Such techniques are very helpful in dealing with noisy data, data scarcity, and for robust model development. Techniques such as GANs, VAEs, and diffusion models enable the learning of complex data distributions from real neural recordings and the generation of new, realistic samples.

#### 6.2.1.1 Generative Adversarial Networks

GANs consist of a generator $G(z)$, which maps latent variables $z$, typically sampled from a simple distribution to synthetic data samples, and a discriminator

**Table 6.1** Applications of generative AI in neural interfaces.

| Application area | Generative technique | Function | Use cases |
|---|---|---|---|
| Synthetic neural data generation | GANs, VAEs, diffusion models | Learn and replicate statistical properties of neural data distributions | Simulating EEG/MEG for training, benchmarking algorithms, rare-condition modeling |
| Data augmentation for model training | Conditional GANs, VAEs, and style-transfer-based models | Enrich training datasets with synthetic samples to improve generalization | Balancing imbalanced datasets, increasing robustness to noise and variability |
| Generative design of neural stimulation patterns | GANs, RL-based generators, VAEs, policy networks | Generate optimized stimulation waveforms for desired neural or motor outcomes | Closed-loop neurostimulation, adaptive neuroprosthetics, therapy personalization |
| Brain-to-text/ Brain-to-image generation | Transformer models, diffusion models, cross-modal encoders | Translate neural signals into structured output in another modality | Decoding imagined speech to text, reconstructing visual imagery from brain activity |

$D(x)$, which attempts to distinguish between real and synthetic samples. Training is framed as a minimax game:

$$\min_{G}\max_{D} \mathbb{E}_{x\sim p_{\text{data}}}[\log D(x)] + \mathbb{E}_{z\sim p(z)}[\log(1 - D(G(z)))].$$

In the context of BCIs, $x$ may represent segments of EEG, ECoG, or fNIRS signals, and $G$ is trained to generate realistic neural time series or feature vectors. Variants such as Wasserstein GANs and conditional GANs (cGANs) often improve stability and allow generation of signals conditioned on labels.

#### 6.2.1.2 Variational Autoencoders

VAEs are generative models that learn a probabilistic latent representation of data. They consist of:

- An encoder $q_\phi(z \mid x)$ approximating the posterior over latent variables.
- A decoder $p_\theta(x \mid z)$ reconstructing data from latent codes.

The VAE is trained by maximizing the evidence lower bound (ELBO):

$$\mathcal{L}_{\text{ELBO}} = \mathbb{E}_{q_\phi(z|x)}[\log p_\theta(x \mid z)] - \text{KL}\big(q_\phi(z \mid x) \parallel p(z)\big),$$

where KL is the Kullback–Leibler divergence.

For BCIs, VAEs can learn smooth latent spaces capturing variability in neural signals across conditions, subjects, or time. Sampling from the latent space of VAEs can generate synthetic signals that match the training distribution, while interpolations in latent space can reveal continuous transitions between neural states.

#### 6.2.1.3 Diffusion Models

Diffusion-based generative models iteratively transform noise into structured samples through a learned denoising process. A forward diffusion process progressively corrupts data with noise, and a neural network is trained to reverse this process step by step. Although quite a computationally demanding, diffusion models can produce high-fidelity samples and have been explored for generating time series and spectrogram-like representations. For neural signals, diffusion models could capture fine-grained temporal structure and variability in oscillatory patterns.

### 6.2.2 Data Augmentation for Model Robustness

Generative models can be used to augment training sets with synthetic samples, addressing data scarcity and class imbalance:

- *Class-conditional generation:* cGANs and conditional VAEs can generate neural data for specific classes such as left vs. right MI, low vs. high workload and also can help to balance classes in datasets for better model learning.
- *Style-transfer augmentation:* These models can generate data representing one condition (a specific user or recording session) in the "style" of another, therefore enabling cross-subject or cross-session augmentation.
- *Noise-aware augmentation:* Generative models can inject realistic noise patterns or simulate specific artifacts, helping classifiers become robust to real-world contamination.

It is important to consider that data augmentation techniques may not produce very accurate data and may also introduce biases which may lead the model to overfit. Therefore, if reporting data using synthetic data, the evaluation metric should include information like similarity measures, performance gains on held-out real data as well as information from the qualitative inspection by domain experts.

### 6.2.3 Generative Design of Neural Stimulation Patterns

Generative AI can also enable the automatic design of neural stimulation protocols, which are critical in applications such as neuroprosthetics, neuromodulation therapies, and sensory feedback systems. Instead of relying on hand-tuned stimulation parameters, generative models can learn to optimize stimulation patterns for specific physiological or behavioral outcomes.

#### 6.2.3.1 Stimulation Pattern Generators

Given a dataset of stimulation patterns $u_t$ and resulting responses like motor outputs, perceived intensity, and neural activity, models can learn mappings:

$$z \mapsto u_t(z) \mapsto \text{response},$$

where $z$ is a latent code capturing desired properties of the response.

- GAN-based generators can propose desired stimulation waveforms, with a discriminator (or separate critic) evaluating efficacy.
- VAEs can provide a structured latent space in which nearby points correspond to similar existing stimulation patterns, facilitating interpolation and exploration.
- RL-based policy networks can directly output stimulation commands based on online feedback, that maximizes the reward function based on brain signals related to cognitive performance.

#### 6.2.3.2 Closed-loop Optimization

In closed-loop setups, stimulation can be adapted in real time based on ongoing neural and behavioral measurements. Generative models can:

- Propose stimulation patterns conditioned on the current brain state, decoded intent, predicted neural evolution, or uncertainty estimates from the decoder. This enables proactive control, especially in rapidly-changing tasks.
- Learn individualized mappings for each subject, capturing idiosyncratic response properties such as nonlinearities, latency effects, or stimulation-dependent neural plasticity. These personalized mapping can allow rapid adaptation without extensive manual tuning.
- Integrate constraints such as safety threshold, stimulation tolerability, or clinical boundaries directly into the generative process to ensure that proposed interventions remain feasible in real-world applications.
- Model the underlying dynamics of brain–stimulation interactions using latent-variable or probabilistic frameworks, enabling prediction of longer-term effects such as habituation. This supports adaptive control policies that optimize performance over extended sessions.

- Provide uncertainty-aware recommendations by representing distributions over possible stimulation parameters, allowing the system to balance exploration by testing new configuration and exploit known effective patterns. This is particularly useful when the neural response is noisy or nonstationary.
- Facilitate RL-based closed-loop optimization by serving as world models or simulators by minimizing the need for direct interaction with the user for every update.
- Allow multi-objective optimization by generating stimulation patterns that jointly optimize accuracy, stability, comfort, latency, or subjective user effort, depending on the goals of the BCI system.

Such systems hold promise for personalized neurostimulation in movement disorders, depression, epilepsy, and sensory augmentation.

### 6.2.4 Multimodal Brain-to-text and Brain-to-image Generation

There is an emerging class of BCIs: brain-to-text and brain-to-image, that allow decoding neural activity for speech and image output. In these BCIs, generative AI plays an important role in learning associated patterns from brain signals to reconstruct and generate linguistic or visual content.

#### 6.2.4.1 Brain-to-text

Brain-to-text systems aim to reconstruct linguistic content directly from neural activity, enabling the decoding of perceived, imagined, or attempted speech. A typical system consists of a neural encoder that transforms ECoG, EEG, fMRI, or intracortical signals into a latent representation $h$, together with a language decoder often a transformer-based language model that generates text conditioned on this latent state. The encoder may employ temporal convolution, recurrent dynamics, or transformer architectures to capture hierarchical linguistic structure, while conditioning of the language model can occur through mechanisms such as cross-attention, prefix tuning, or prompting that modulates its hidden states.

Training relies on paired neural–linguistic datasets in which neural recordings are aligned with speech, auditory stimuli, or internal narration. The objective function combines token-level cross-entropy for text generation with alignment losses, such as connectionist temporal classification (CTC) and temporal contrastive objectives to help associate neural time series with phonemes, syllables, or semantic segments. Additional embedding-level or semantic consistency losses encourage the latent neural representation to align with the representation spaces of pretrained language models.

More advanced brain-to-text system introduces intermediate decoding stages such as neural-to-phoneme or articulatory decoding to improve robustness when data are limited. Other extensions support zero-shot or few-shot generalization by aligning neural features with pretrained language model embeddings, or incorporate uncertainty-aware decoding strategies that provide probabilistic estimates reflecting ambiguity in neural activity.

#### 6.2.4.2 Brain-to-image

Brain-to-image systems aim to reconstruct or approximate visual content directly from neural activity, providing a means to infer perceptual or imagined imagery from brain signals. Such systems typically pair a neural encoder, which maps fMRI activation patterns, EEG-derived features, or ECoG signals into a latent representation, with a visual generative model that produces images conditioned on this latent space. The encoder may employ spatial feature extraction, voxel-to-latent regression, or manifold-alignment techniques to match neural features to the internal representation of the generative model. The generative component is often instantiated as a diffusion model, GAN, VAE, or multimodal vision–language decoder that reconstructs images from latent vectors or conditioning embeddings.

Recent approaches increasingly leverage joint vision–language model spaces, such as contrastive language-image pre-training (CLIP), to align brain-derived representations with semantic image embeddings. In these systems, neural signals are mapped into a shared latent space where semantic similarity guides reconstruction, and the generative model uses this representation to refine visual features through iterative denoising or latent optimization. Training objectives include reconstruction losses, cross-modal alignment losses between neural and image embeddings, and regularization terms encouraging consistency with the generative model's latent manifold. Diffusion-based pipelines further incorporate neural conditioning into each denoising step, enabling high-fidelity reconstructions that capture both structural features and higher-level semantics of the underlying visual content.

## 6.3 From Decoding to Intelligent Interaction

ML and generative AI together enable a progression from basic neural decoding to rich, intelligent interaction. Classical supervised and unsupervised methods provide foundational tools for mapping features to labels and discovering latent structure in neural data. DL architectures enhance this capability by learning hierarchical representations and capturing complex spatiotemporal dependencies, while RL and transfer learning support continual adaptation to changing users and environments.

Generative AI extends the role of neural interfaces beyond classification and regression. By synthesizing realistic neural data, augmenting training sets, generating stimulation patterns, and translating neural activity into text, images, or avatar behavior, generative models transform BCIs into expressive, creative, and highly personalized systems. In closed-loop architectures, decoded intent, generative outputs, and adaptive control policies can be combined to form interactive agents that co-evolve with the user, continually optimizing both performance and subjective experience.

## 6.4 Summary

This chapter has examined the role of ML and generative AI in neural interfaces. It has provided an overview of supervised and unsupervised learning methods for neural data analysis, highlighting classical classifiers, clustering, and dimensionality reduction techniques. It then discussed DL architectures such as CNNs, RNNs, LSTMs, and transformers, which learn hierarchical and temporally aware representations from high-dimensional neural signals. RL and transfer learning were presented as key frameworks for adaptive and personalized BCIs, enabling systems to adjust to user feedback and reduce calibration effort.

The chapter further explored the growing applications of generative AI in neural interfaces, including synthetic neural data generation, data augmentation, generative design of stimulation patterns, and brain-to-text and brain-to-image translation. These approaches extend neural interfaces from passive decoding devices to active, creative collaborators capable of simulating, augmenting, and expressing neural states in rich multimodal forms.

Together with the automated signal processing foundations presented in the previous chapter, the methods discussed here provide the algorithmic backbone for next-generation BCI systems that are robust, adaptive, scalable, and capable of supporting natural, continuous, and highly personalized interaction in real-world settings.

# 7

# Innovative Environment and Tools

The development of effective brain–computer interface (BCI) systems is significantly dependent on a comprehensive ecosystem of environments, tools, and methodologies that support the design, implementation, and evaluation of experiments and applications. Over recent years, the BCI research community has explored a number of innovative approaches to improve accessibility, adaptability, and robustness of BCI technologies. These approaches are based on interactive paradigms inspired from game design, immersive virtual and augmented reality (VR/AR) environments, portable at-home experimental setups, and modular development toolkits. Such tools and methods are not only driving technical progress but also reshaping the way BCI experiments are conceived, deployed, and experienced across academic, clinical, and consumer domains. The inherently interdisciplinary nature of BCI research is situated at the intersection of neuroscience, engineering, computer science, and psychology and requires development environments that are equally versatile. A BCI system required real-time neural signal acquisition, adaptive feedback mechanisms, multimodal data integration, and user-centric interaction design. Whether the goal is to implement a neurofeedback game, embed a cognitive task within a VR scenario, or conduct a longitudinal behavioral study remotely, current BCI development relies on a diverse software and hardware toolkit that goes far beyond basic data collection. Integration of experimental protocols, signal processing pipelines, user interfaces, and platform interoperability is essential for scalable, reproducible, and innovative BCI research.

As the field continues to grow toward real-world BCI applications and broader accessibility, the focus has expanded from algorithmic performance to improving user experience, system portability, and ease of integration. This effort is required to make BCI systems that require minimal hardware setup times, are capable of wireless and mobile operation, streamline experimental design, and are able to incorporate additional modalities such as eye tracking and motion capture. In this context, the design of the BCI development environment itself plays a critical role. A well-constructed environment can help to mitigate cognitive fatigue, enhance signal quality, and support more intuitive and engaging user interactions. This chapter provides a detailed overview of the evolving landscape of BCI development environments and tools. It examines the motivation introduced through gamified tasks, the sensory and spatial engagement by immersive mixed reality (MR) platforms, and the democratization of BCI research through portable and take-home kits. It also explores the role of key development frameworks such as Unity, OpenVibe, and Lab Streaming Layer (LSL), which are essential for rapid prototyping and real-time experimentation.

## 7.1 Gamified Environment

Gamification refers to the use of game design elements such as points, levels, challenges, and rewards in non-gaming contexts. In the context-specific applications, the gamified environment is also known as game with the purpose (GWAP) or Serious Gaming [81]. Gamification is very common in cognitive neuroscience experiments, which are used to create neural correlates of different cognitive functions. In addition to this, gamification is also very useful for improving motivation, user engagement, and learning outcomes. Let us look closely how gamified environment making difference for BCIs development.

### 7.1.1 Game Mechanics for BCI Engagement

Game mechanics in BCI engagement aim to bridge the gap between cognitive effort and interactive feedback. These mechanics do not simply make tasks entertaining, but they serve as structured components that help sustain attention, motivate learning, and provide measurable outcomes. Some of the most commonly used mechanics in BCI games include:

- Point systems: These reward users with visual or numerical scores based on the quality of their brain signals.
- Real-time feedback: Providing immediate visual or auditory cues that reflect ongoing brain activity, helping users learn control over time. In BCI context, real-time feedback sometimes also refers to neurofeedback.
- Progressive difficulty: Increasing the challenge as user performance improves to maintain engagement and prevent boredom.
- Time-limited challenges: These add time pressure to increase cognitive load and simulate realistic task conditions.
- Unlockable content or levels: Motivating long-term use by allowing users to unlock new environments or tasks as they master previous ones.

- Narrative-driven design: Embedding BCI tasks in a story context to give users a sense of progression and purpose.
- Exploration-based progression: This allows users to discover new elements or areas through successful brain-controlled actions, therefore reinforcing curiosity and reward-seeking behavior.
- Social competition: This is a relatively advanced version of gamification where multiplayer BCI setups may allow users to compete or collaborate using brain signals, increasing motivation and engagement.

Despite their benefits, these advanced mechanics require careful and thoughtful implementation. A common risk of such mechanics is overstimulation by introducing too many visual elements or delivering feedback at a pace that overwhelms the user. Such a condition could lead to distraction and degrade the quality of brain signals. Another well-known concern is cognitive fatigue. It is becoming a growing and a serious concern when tasks are not well-balanced. Balancing these considerations is key to developing BCI experiences that are both engaging and scientifically valid with gamification.

### 7.1.2 Adaptive Difficulty

Adaptive difficulty in BCI systems refers to the dynamic adjustment of task challenge levels based on the user's real-time performance or cognitive state. This is a relatively advanced way to improve engagement within gamification mechanics. Such systems continuously tailor the task to maintain an optimal zone of engagement. By doing so. it stimulates learning and helps to produce effective BCI-related brain signals while not being so difficult that it leads to frustration or fatigue. Adaptive difficulty mechanisms respond to this by monitoring key performance indicators such as:

- Classification accuracy: Tracking the success rate of brain signal interpretation in real time.
- Signal strength and consistency: This evaluates whether brain activity remains stable and within target frequency ranges.
- Reaction time or task completion speed: It uses timing metrics as indirect indicators of mental effort or fatigue.
- Engagement level: Inferred from electroencephalography (EEG) patterns or behavioral data, such as task abandonment or reduced interaction.

These indicators are used to adjust the complexity of the task in real time. For example, in a BCI game using motor imagery (MI), if high accuracy is detected consistently, the system might increase task difficulty by reducing time limits, adding distractors, or introducing multi-step goals. If the performance drops below a threshold, the task may simplify itself by offering longer decision windows, visual aids, or more forgiving scoring criteria. Although adaptive difficulty improves user engagement and personalization in BCI systems, it also introduces a number of design and implementation challenges. The very mechanisms that make adaptive systems responsive and flexible can also lead to unpredictability, data inconsistency, or unintended cognitive effects if not properly managed. Adaptive systems must also be carefully validated to ensure they are not reinforcing undesirable strategies or overfitting to short-term performance patterns.

Table 7.1 shows a summary for different gamification strategies in BCI as well as what to consider before using them.

**Table 7.1** Summary of gamification strategies in BCI systems.

| Gamification element | Function | Considerations |
|---|---|---|
| **Point systems** | Provide measurable feedback and reinforce performance using brain signals | Risk of over-reliance on extrinsic motivation; may need calibration to avoid discouragement |
| **Real-time feedback** | Help users learn self-regulation of brain activity; close the feedback loop in real time | Overcomplex visuals and audio can overstimulate and distract, degrading signal quality |
| **Progressive difficulty** | Maintain challenge as performance improves; prevent engagement plateau | Difficulty curve must be well-balanced to avoid cognitive overload or boredom |
| **Time-limited challenges** | Increase cognitive load, simulate time pressure for realistic scenarios | Can cause stress or fatigue; not suitable for all user profiles |
| **Progress levels** | Encourage long-term engagement and mastery of control strategies | Requires thoughtful reward pacing; must align with user goals |
| **Narrative-driven** | Provide purpose, immersion, and progression through storytelling | Risk of narrative elements overshadowing task clarity or focus |
| **Exploration-based progression** | Reinforce curiosity and reward-driven brain activity | May require more complex control strategies, impacting accessibility |
| **Social competition** | Leverage peer dynamics to enhance motivation and engagement | Multiplayer setups introduce synchronization and fairness challenges |
| **Adaptive difficulty** | Dynamically optimize task challenge based on user performance or state | Needs careful calibration; may reinforce undesirable strategies or overfit to noise |

### 7.1.3 Studies of Game-based BCI Applications

Game-based BCI applications have been widely explored across research, clinical, and educational settings, serving as powerful testbeds for real-time BCIs. These applications combine entertainment value with functional purpose, enabling users to control or influence game environments using only brain activities. While the mechanics vary, the goal is often consistent to create an engaging, adaptive, and measurable system that encourages neural learning, rehabilitation, control, or performance tracking. There are several notable BCI paradigms where gamification is introduced and successful.

#### 7.1.3.1 MI Training Through Racing Games

One of the most widely explored applications of gamification in BCI research is the use of racing games controlled by MI. In these scenarios, user imagines limb movements such as left or right-hand movement, which modulate sensorimotor rhythms in the mu (8–12 Hz) and beta (13–30 Hz) bands over the motor cortex. These neural signals are then decoded in real time to control the direction or speed of a racing avatar or vehicle.

- Such games are very common in stroke rehabilitation research, where they offer engaging alternatives to repetitive physical exercises for motor relearning
- Performance feedback is provided in real time through visual or auditory cues, helping users adjust their mental strategies and gradually gain better control over their neural signals.
- Studies [82] report significantly higher user motivation and task adherence compared to traditional BCI calibration tasks, leading to faster adaptation to MI protocols and better long-term training outcomes.
- Some systems [83] incorporate adaptive difficulty, progressively increasing challenge as the user's motor control improves, ensuring continued cognitive and neural engagement throughout the training.

These games not only serve therapeutic goals but also help establish intuitive mental strategies through engaging, real-time feedback. The integration of reward-based progression (e.g., laps completed, speed boosts) aligns closely with game design principles, making MI training more approachable for both clinical and healthy users.

#### 7.1.3.2 Attention Monitoring in First-person Navigation Games

First-person navigation games provide an innovative framework for monitoring and training attention based on real-time EEG signals [84]. These games use neural markers such as increased frontal theta activity or reduced parietal alpha power to estimate the user's attentional state, which is then used to modulate the game environment dynamically.

- These systems continuously monitor extracted features from brain signals correlated with sustained attention and vigilance, adjusting in-game behavior based on these markers.
- If inattention is detected, the game may slow down movement, introduce penalties, or distort visuals, encouraging the user to regain focus to proceed effectively.
- Real-time adaptive feedback trains users to self-regulate attention by maintaining high engagement levels, making these games useful for populations with attentional deficits such as ADHD [85].
- Some designs incorporate distractions or dynamic environments to simulate real-world challenges, helping assess and train attention in ecologically valid scenarios.

By embedding attention regulation into immersive gameplay, such applications combine neurofeedback training with interaction. They also provide a testbed for evaluating attentional load, vigilance decrement, and user response to cognitive challenges in controlled but realistic settings.

#### 7.1.3.3 Neurofeedback Through Puzzle and Memory Games

Puzzle and memory-based games integrated with neurofeedback mechanisms are frequently used to train cognitive skills such as working memory, sustained attention, and mental flexibility. These games are commonly developed using EEG-based features reflecting cognitive load, engagement, or error processing and adapt dynamically to support learning.

- Neurofeedback can be delivered through in-game mechanics such as changing colors, animated effects, or auditory tones, which reflect the user's cognitive state in a non-intrusive way.
- Users learn to voluntarily modulate their brain states, such as calming down when over-aroused or focusing when distracted, by interpreting and responding to these feedback cues.
- Longitudinal studies show improvements in task accuracy and reaction time, as well as positive transfer effects on unrelated cognitive tasks outside the game context.
- These games are particularly suited for educational, aging, or cognitive rehabilitation populations where structured cognitive training is needed.

The structure of these games encourages iterative learning cycles, where users receive immediate neural feedback and adjust their mental strategy accordingly.

This dynamic interplay between brain state and game mechanics enhances both cognitive training efficacy and user satisfaction.

#### 7.1.3.4 Social Interaction in Multiplayer Games

Multiplayer BCI games [86, 87] represent an emerging area where users interact cooperatively or competitively using their brain signals as input. Such systems introduce a social layer to BCI interaction, which is based on the motivational benefits of peer engagement and competition while exploring novel aspects of shared cognitive control.

- In cooperative scenarios, players may be required to synchronize their brain signals, also known as hyperscanning, to achieve shared goals such as opening a locked door or navigating a complex task together.
- These applications open up new possibilities in studying BCI-based social synchrony, empathy, and collaboration, which are relevant in affective neuroscience and multiuser communication studies.
- Competitive formats have also been explored, where brain-based performance metrics are used to determine winners. This adds game theoretic dynamics and helps to motivate users through rivalry.
- The inclusion of social interaction adds realism and complexity to BCI systems, therefore making them closer to real-life communication and teamwork situations.

Multiplayer BCIs require synchronization of data streams and feedback mechanisms. However, they offer a platform for exploring inter-brain dynamics and cooperative neurofeedback applications, potentially useful in social cognition therapies or training environments.

#### 7.1.3.5 Emotional Regulation Games Using Affective BCI

Affective BCI systems seek to identify and respond to users' emotional states by decoding neural features associated with affect, such as frontal alpha asymmetry or changes in theta and beta band activity. Games based on these systems provide interactive feedback based on emotional regulation and can offer environments suitable for emotional training.

- In affective games, players influence the game environment based on their emotional balance. For example, a tranquil virtual garden may flourish when the user remains calm but degrade under high emotional arousal.
- Environmental elements such as weather, lighting, music, and object interaction are dynamically altered based on emotional state, creating a direct brain-emotion-game feedback loop.

- These games train users in emotional self-regulation, making them useful in applications such as anxiety reduction, mindfulness practice, and resilience training.
- Some systems include guided breathing, meditation elements, or narrative storytelling to support relaxation and long-term emotional awareness.

These affective games are particularly relevant in therapeutic, educational, and mental health contexts. They combine biofeedback principles with immersive interaction, discussed more in detail in next section, which allows users to explore and train emotional awareness and stability in a highly personalized and engaging format.

## 7.2 AR, VR, and MR Environment

VR is a technology that creates an artificial and simulated environment where users are fully immersed and visually separated from the physical world. In BCI applications, VR provides a highly controlled virtual space suitable for implementing experimental protocols, training regimens, and neurofeedback paradigms. VR can be used in combination with brain signals where these signals can be detected in real time and translated into commands for tasks such as spatial navigation, object manipulation, or avatar control. For example, users can perform MI tasks to control the movement of a virtual hand in three-dimensional space, while the system interprets corresponding changes in sensorimotor rhythms. Due to the highly controlled virtual environment, VR systems also allow dynamic adaptation of task parameters and provide visual feedback by changing the surrounding virtual environment, like colors, scenes, and sounds, in response to engagement levels, thereby improving user motivation and supporting sustained learning. Such interactions have been seen to significantly accelerate rehabilitation among users and improve mental health and wellbeing.

AR provides an environment by superimposing digital elements on the real world. These elements could be instructions, graphical indicators, virtual buttons, or data. Similar to VR, brain signals in AR enable the selection or manipulation of these digital overlays. For instance, neural markers of visual attention such as P300 can be used to select among multiple visible options, or steady-state visually evoked potentials (SSVEP) may be overlaid on physical objects to trigger actions based on user intent. Because AR allows users to remain aware of their surroundings while interacting with virtual overlay elements, it is particularly well suited to mobile real-world BCI applications, smart environment control, and assistive technologies.

MR is an extension of the functionality of both VR and AR, while also allowing contextual and spatial awareness. It allows users to interact with both virtual and physical objects, where virtual objects also interact with the real world in the same shared space. For example, users can fly a virtual drone which lands on real tables using cognitive effort, providing a direct mapping between internal neural states and external outcomes.

The growing availability of commercial head-mounted displays, including HTC Vive, Apple Vision Pro, Meta Quest, and Varjo, has accelerated the application of AR, VR, and MR technologies beyond controlled laboratory settings. These devices also provide real-time motion tracking and bio-physical sensing such as facial expression, hand, and eye tracking. Importantly, they also allow integration with development platforms like Lab Streaming Layer (LSL) and popular game engines, therefore enabling deployment in different settings, including take-home therapy, training, and consumer-facing applications. The widespread accessibility of these technologies is supporting their growing importance for the future of BCI systems.

### 7.2.1 Application Scenarios of Immersive BCI Systems

When combined with BCIs, immersive environments based on AR, VR, or MR provide powerful capability for simulating complex cognitive and behavioral tasks. These systems are now used in a variety of application domains ranging from clinical therapy to cognitive research and interactive entertainment.

- **Motor rehabilitation:** BCI systems integrated with VR are used to support motor recovery by enabling patients to engage in MI or attempted movement tasks in immersive virtual environments [88]. These tasks, paired with real-time visual feedback, reinforce activation of motor regions in the brain. MR applications further enrich this experience by allowing users to interact with both physical and virtual objects, supporting fine motor control and skill transfer.
- **Neuroadaptive gaming:** Immersive games powered by BCI leverage neural signals related to attention, emotion, or command-based control. These applications serve as tools for training cognitive functions such as sustained attention or stress management. Games driven by ERPs (such as P300), SSVEPs, or affective states offer a high degree of personalization and engagement, making them suitable for long-term training, evaluation, or even entertainment purposes.
- **Cognitive workload and multitasking:** Immersive environments allow for the presentation of layered stimuli and dynamic task conditions that reflect real-world complexity. BCI systems can monitor neural signatures of cognitive load in real time, adjusting task difficulty or timing to maintain an optimal engagement level. Such applications are particularly relevant in domains like aviation, driving, and adaptive human–computer interaction.

An emerging trend in immersive BCI research is the integration of additional physiological signals, such as heart rate, skin conductance, respiration, and electromyography, along with neural data from EEG, fNIRS, or invasive implants. Of particular importance is the use of eye-tracking technology, which offers continuous and unobtrusive access to gaze behavior, attentional patterns, and visual engagement. When combined with neural signals, these data streams provide a multidimensional profile of user state, enhancing both system responsiveness and interpretability.

- **Eye tracking:** Provides real-time insights into user attention, gaze fixation, and visual behavior, complementing EEG-based assessments of cognitive engagement.
- **Facial expression:** Captures subtle facial muscle activations through cameras or EMG sensors, enabling detection of facial action units and enriching multimodal user-state estimation.
- **Haptic feedback:** Enables the delivery of tactile stimuli that support immersive learning and sensorimotor integration, especially in rehabilitation contexts.
- **Voice and motion capture:** Facilitate natural interaction in mixed environments, enabling gesture-based commands and vocal responses to be integrated with brain signal input.

The convergence of neural, physiological, and behavioral data within immersive platforms is enabling the development of highly adaptive BCI systems. Such systems provide nuanced control, personalization, and improved interpretability, which are essential for real-world deployment across clinical, educational, and entertainment domains.

## 7.3 Take-home Experiments

Take-home experiments in BCI research are an emerging area of interest, which is supported by recent advancements in portable neural recording technologies and compact artificial intelligence (AI) models. Although to fully realized these systems for in-home experimentation are still in developmental stages, early efforts are demonstrating the potential to extend cognitive neuroscience research beyond traditional laboratory settings. The use of portable EEG, fNIRS, and other wearable systems have shown feasibility to investigate cognitive and neural phenomena in more natural environments.

The take-home experiment paradigm envisions a framework in which users can participate in longitudinal or adaptive research protocols while embedded in their everyday routines. These studies hold promise for capturing how cognitive states and brain activity unfold in real-world conditions, enabling researchers to examine a variety of cognitive and behavioral factors which shape natural cognition.

### 7.3.1 Remote and Longitudinal Research

As the field moves toward more distributed and user-centered research paradigms, there is increasing interest in the development of BCI systems that are suitable for remote and longitudinal studies. These systems are expected to be compact, wireless, and equipped with intuitive user interfaces, often supported by mobile applications or web-based platforms. In such systems, participants are guided through structured protocols remotely, with automated logging and adaptive feedback tailored to individual progress. Although very few prototyped systems currently exist (see this review [89]), the anticipated advantages of remote BCI research are numerous. Long-term data collection can facilitate the study of learning effects, neuroplasticity, and behavioral adaptation across days or weeks. Areas such as sleep research, cognitive decline monitoring, mental health tracking, and rehabilitation could particularly benefit from this approach. Data captured in naturalistic settings can also provide new insights into how brain dynamics are shaped by everyday environmental and social contexts, therefore minimizing the artificiality commonly imposed by controlled laboratory experiments.

### 7.3.2 Home-based Cognitive and Motor Experiments

Emerging prototypes of home-based experimental platforms suggest promising applications in domains such as cognitive monitoring, motor rehabilitation, and adaptive learning. In an ideal setting, patients recovering from motor impairments could engage in guided MI exercises or neurofeedback training at home, therefore reducing the frequency of hospital visits and improving long-term adherence. Similarly, students might engage with gamified, brain-driven educational content in natural settings, providing researchers with extended neural data tied to engagement and retention. Potential applications under exploration include the monitoring of attention span during daily activities and tracking of cognitive workload during multitasking tasks performed in real-life environments. In these contexts, wearable BCI technology could support unobtrusive and flexible data collection, while AI-driven systems provide automated quality assurance and user feedback.

Despite their promise, take-home experiments introduce several technical and methodological challenges, especially with noninvasive devices such as:

- High susceptibility to signal noise due to uncontrolled recording environments
- Improper electrode placement or device calibration by unsupervised users
- Limited protocol adherence and task consistency in the absence of direct supervision

### 7.3.3 Usability and Compliance in Unsupervised Settings

One of the main limitations of early BCI systems was their complexity, which required expert technicians for setup and calibration. However, recent advancements in hardware such as dry electrodes, wearable EEG and fNIRS headsets, and integrated signal amplifiers have made BCI more accessible for non-expert users for take-home setups. This includes simplified calibration procedures, mobile-guided interfaces, and automatic syncing of data to cloud platforms. These features significantly improve existing take-home challenges and user compliance in unsupervised environments. To support user adherence over time, some systems can include:

- Daily reminders or task scheduling notifications
- Interactive tutorials and progress feedback
- Gamified scoring and achievement tracking

These design strategies not only improve compliance but also maintain user engagement throughout the experiment duration.

### 7.3.4 Examples of Real-world Deployment

Several research studies and commercial pilot programs have successfully demonstrated the viability of take-home BCI systems. Below we examine two leading modalities: EEG and fNIRS with representative real-world take-home studies.

#### 7.3.4.1 EEG-based Take-home Experiments

Portable EEG headsets have been widely deployed in real-life settings. In sleep research, users wore EEG headbands over multiple nights, and the data supported the validation of at-home sleep trackers, showing reliable recording of sleep stages comparable to clinical polysomnography [90]. In cognitive training, participants with multiple sclerosis performed neurofeedback over home use (ten sessions in 3–4 weeks), which led to improved attention and memory, as well as detectable white-matter and functional connectivity changes on MRI [91]. Similarly, a home-based neurofeedback pilot in neuropathic pain patients used an eight-week protocol with portable EEG, yielding reduced pain and improved mood [92]. Another feasibility study with Parkinson's disease patients demonstrated that at-home EEG neurofeedback helped participants learn to self-regulate mu rhythms, enhancing motor response onset [93].

#### 7.3.4.2 fNIRS-based Take-home Experiments

Wearable fNIRS devices have emerged as powerful tools for at-home brain monitoring. In a pilot work [94], motor cortex lateralization was measured in 11 chronic stroke survivors using a wireless fNIRS headband during upper limb exercises performed at home. Lateralization indices correlated strongly with both impairment and functional status, validating the system's feasibility outside laboratory settings [95]. Separately, a consumer-grade Mendi fNIRS reading taken at home during a Stroop task has been compared to those acquired in the lab via Biopac; the devices exhibited high concordance (group-level $r \approx 0.81$) [96]. Moreover, a 2023 validation confirmed that a two-channel Mendi headset captured cognitive load-dependent prefrontal oxygenation changes during n-back tasks, demonstrating sensitivity to working memory load in take-home contexts. Other developments include wireless, fiberless fNIRS headbands that perform comparably to full-cap systems in detecting sensorimotor activity [97], and novel open-source platforms such as OpenNIRScap, a 24-channel low-cost wearable fNIRS cap suitable for real-time cognitive monitoring in everyday settings [98].

Together, take-home EEG and fNIRS systems demonstrate that high-quality neural biomarkers, which range from sleep cycles and cognitive load to motor cortex asymmetry. These neural biomarkers can be measured reliably outside the laboratory. These studies underscore home-based BCIs' potential in enabling personalized rehabilitation, cognitive enhancement, and longitudinal health monitoring.

### 7.3.5 Popular Tools and Frameworks for BCI Development

Developing reliable, real-time BCI requires robust software environments that support multimodal data acquisition, automated signal processing, and adaptive information generation. There are several software tools that facilitate prototyping and BCI development by allowing remote operation, hardware abstraction, synchronization, and user-friendly deployment. This section provides an overview of widely used platforms for BCI development and applications.

#### 7.3.5.1 Unity: Game Engine

Unity [99] is a cross-platform game engine that has become popular in the BCI community for creating immersive, interactive environments not just for PC and mobile applications but also AR/VR and MR environments. Unity allows building neurofeedback training games, adaptive user interfaces, and experimental paradigms in cognitive neuroscience. Unity provides real-time rendering capabilities and seamless integration with external application programming interfaces (APIs) and hardware.

For BCI applications, Unity can receive neurophysiological inputs (e.g., EEG, fNIRS) via communication protocols such as LSL or through middleware like BrainFlow. Researchers can map signal features such as attention levels or motor intentions to game parameters or visual stimuli, enabling real-time closed-loop systems.

#### 7.3.5.2 OpenVibe: Modular Signal Processing Platform

OpenVibe [100] is an open-source, graph-based software environment for the development and testing of BCI applications. It provides a visual programming interface to design signal acquisition, preprocessing including filtering, and artifact removal, feature extraction, classification, and feedback presentation pipelines. OpenVibe is particularly suitable for prototyping novel BCI paradigms without requiring extensive programming expertise. It supports a variety of EEG hardware through built-in drivers and is often used for MI, P300 spellers, and attention-monitoring studies. Its open architecture also allows integration with external engines such as Unity for real-time stimulus control. Although traditionally used in lab-based research, OpenVibe has also been adapted for portable BCI systems by embedding its engine into lightweight devices or using it in conjunction with mobile data acquisition modules.

#### 7.3.5.3 BCI2000: General-purpose BCI Development System

BCI2000 [101] is a mature, extensible software framework for real-time BCI research. Developed at the Wadsworth Center (USA), it is designed for clinical and experimental use. Its modular architecture includes components for data acquisition, signal processing, user feedback, and logging. BCI2000 supports a wide array of EEG hardware and has been used in numerous clinical trials and neurorehabilitation protocols, including stroke recovery and communication aids for individuals with severe motor impairment. It also supports integration with custom scripts and external applications. Although it was initially built for lab environments, recent efforts have explored its real-world deployment, especially for longitudinal studies in assistive BCI.

#### 7.3.5.4 NeuroPype: Modular Real-time BCI Framework

NeuroPype [102] is a commercial platform designed for real-time signal processing and BCI development. It adopts a flow-based programming model, enabling users to build signal processing pipelines using a drag-and-drop interface. NeuroPype supports multimodal data inputs, including EEG, eye tracking, galvanic skin response (GSR), and heart rate, making it a powerful tool for affective computing and neuroadaptive interfaces. NeuroPype is well-suited for take-home BCI experimentation due to its integrated support for remote data acquisition, cloud synchronization, and compatibility with consumer EEG devices. It is frequently used for neurofeedback training, workload assessment, and human–computer interaction research. The platform also allows Python-based scripting for advanced users.

#### 7.3.5.5 Simulink and MATLAB for Real-time BCI Prototyping

Simulink [103], a part of the MATLAB ecosystem, provides a graphical environment for modeling, simulating, and implementing real-time systems. In BCI research, it is commonly used for developing signal processing pipelines, machine learning classifiers, and real-time feedback mechanisms. With toolboxes such as the signal processing toolbox and neural network toolbox, Simulink allows researchers to rapidly prototype and evaluate algorithms before deploying them in embedded or mobile systems. Simulink Real-Time and xPC Target enable low-latency applications. Integration with LSL and hardware APIs, researchers can build closed-loop neurofeedback or motor-control systems that operate reliably even outside of lab conditions.

Table 7.2 lists a summary for all the popular tools and their primary user and suitability for BCI application, especially in real-world environment.

**Table 7.2** Overview of common BCI software platforms and their suitability for real-time BCI systems.

| Platform | Type | Primary use case | Suitability |
|---|---|---|---|
| **Unity** | Game engine/ interface environment | Creation of immersive feedback systems and training games using EEG or fNIRS inputs | High; supports real-time interactive neurofeedback in cognitive training, rehabilitation and also suitable to AR/VR/MR development |
| **OpenVibe** | Modular signal processing platform | Visual design of BCI pipelines: acquisition, filtering, classification, feedback | Moderate; adaptable for portable EEG but requires adaptation for mobile deployment |
| **BCI2000** | General-purpose BCI framework | Clinical and research BCIs for motor imagery, P300, and neuroprosthetics | Moderate; well-established in clinical use, emerging home-based applications |
| **NeuroPype** | Commercial modular framework | Real-time EEG pipelines with visual programming and multimodal integration | High; optimized for home use and consumer-grade devices, supports cloud features |
| **Simulink** | Real-time modeling and algorithm prototyping tools | Signal processing, machine learning, and system control for BCI | Moderate; powerful but less lightweight, suited for lab-linked mobile BCI setups |

## 7.4 Summary

The development of effective and user-friendly BCI systems depends not only on advances in signal processing or hardware design but also on the broader ecosystem of tools and environments that support their deployment. As explored in this chapter, the BCI field is evolving through the convergence of several innovative approaches that together are reshaping how BCI research is conducted and how applications are designed.

Gamified scenarios introduce structured, motivating, and feedback-rich tasks that are especially useful for training users to generate consistent brain signals. These approaches promote sustained engagement and improve learning outcomes, making BCI more accessible to diverse user groups. At the same time, immersive environments based on VR, AR, and MR offer a flexible and realistic context for interaction, which is critical for applications ranging from cognitive rehabilitation to neuroadaptive gaming. The integration of BCI with these environments allows for dynamic and context-sensitive interaction, resulting in systems that are not only functionally effective but also engaging and ecologically valid.

Take-home experiments, made feasible by portable hardware and intelligent signal processing tools, further extend the reach of BCI research beyond the laboratory. Such systems support long-term and naturalistic data collection, therefore enabling new insights into neural activity during daily life. With the help of AI-based features for signal cleaning, performance feedback, and adaptive task delivery, take-home BCI platforms are becoming robust tools for cognitive assessment, education, and home-based therapy.

There is also growing interest in software tools for the BCI lifecycle, both for experiments and applications. Tools such as Unity, OpenVibe, LSL, BCI2000, EEGLAB, and NeuroPype allow researchers to build modular, scalable, and interoperable systems tailored to specific research goals and applications. The integration of these tools across experimental pipelines enables precise synchronization, advanced analytics, machine learning, classification, and real-time feedback, all of which are essential for developing practical and reliable BCI applications.

In summary, the current generation of tools and environments reflects a shift in BCI research toward real-world relevance, user-centered design, and interdisciplinary collaboration. Such innovations are not only accelerating scientific discovery but also laying the foundation for future BCI systems that are adaptive, immersive, and seamlessly embedded into everyday life.

# 8

# Applications of Brain–Computer Interfaces

The rapid progress across multiple disciplines that contribute to brain–computer interface (BCI) development has made it possible to design and implement a wide variety of applications. These range from clinical interventions to tools intended for use by healthy individuals. Around the world, researchers, developers, and innovative startups are actively pursuing new directions, opening new possibilities that were once considered purely speculative. One of the most dynamic areas of this progress is the race to develop advanced invasive BCI systems. In the sections, we will examine how BCIs are being applied across different fields, exploring the achievements, and future potential of these technologies.

## 8.1 Medical

The initial motivation for developing BCIs largely emerged from the medical field. The primary goal was to assist individuals with physical impairments, particularly those resulting from spinal cord injuries or motor neuron diseases. These conditions often lead to significant loss of motor function, motivating researchers to explore how BCIs could be used to restore some degree of control and independence. Initially, BCI development focused on restoring partial motor function, such as enabling basic limb movement or communication through neural signals. Over time, however, the scope of medical BCI applications has expanded significantly. Today, these systems are not only used to support motor recovery but are also being explored for their potential in cognitive enhancement, neurorehabilitation, diagnosis, and treatment.

In this space, invasive BCIs have shown the greatest promise in restoring motor function, particularly in individuals with spinal cord injuries or neurodegenerative conditions such as Parkinson's disease. Meanwhile, noninvasive systems have proven especially useful in areas related to mental health, including the diagnosis and treatment of psychiatric and neurological disorders. The following are key areas where BCIs are currently applied within the medical domain.

### 8.1.1 Neuroprosthetics

Motor function is one of the most important capabilities of the human body. It plays a central role in enabling autonomy and facilitating interaction with the environment. The ability to perform intentional physical movements is closely tied to an individual's sense of independence and overall quality of life. When this ability is impaired, whether partially or completely due to injury or disease, the consequences are significant. These effects extend not only to the individuals affected but also to their families, caregivers, and the broader healthcare system. To address these challenges, researchers have experimented on developing assistive technologies, particularly neuroprosthetics. These are prosthetic devices that can be directly controlled through neural signals. The goal is to replicate natural limb movements by interpreting signals generated by the brain or peripheral nervous system. BCI has emerged as a key technology in this effort. In particular, MI-based paradigms, which rely on the mental imagination of movement, have demonstrated the ability to produce usable control signals for operating prosthetic limbs.

Invasive BCI approaches, which involve implanting electrodes on the surface of or within the brain, offer high-resolution control by capturing detailed neural activity related to motor planning. Noninvasive approaches, such as those using electroencephalography (EEG) provide limited spatial resolution but still enable meaningful control when supported by sophisticated signal processing techniques. These systems have helped individuals with conditions such as spinal cord injury or limb amputation partially regain functional capabilities. Although still in the development phase, neuroprosthetic applications of BCI technology are progressing toward real-world usability, with several research prototypes demonstrating promising results in clinical and experimental settings.

### 8.1.2 Rehabilitation

Rehabilitation is the therapeutic process of restoring lost or impaired physical functions following neurological damage. This process is most often required after events such as stroke, spinal cord injury, or traumatic brain injury. It typically involves repeated physical exercises conducted under the supervision of medical professionals. These exercises aim to rebuild neural connections and reestablish voluntary control over motor functions. Traditional rehabilitation is labor intensive and often requires long periods of therapy guided by a trained specialist. While these methods are effective, they can be slow and resource demanding. In recent years, BCI has been introduced as a way to enhance and accelerate the rehabilitation process. BCI assisted rehabilitation enables patients to engage in mental or attempted physical activity, and the corresponding brain signals are used to control external devices such as robotic limbs or virtual avatars. This closed loop interaction reinforces neuroplasticity, the brain's ability to adapt and reorganize itself, which is essential for recovery.

MI-based BCI systems are particularly effective in this context. When a patient imagines moving a limb, brain signals associated with that imagined movement are detected and used to activate feedback systems. Over time, this process can help restore the brain's ability to generate and coordinate motor commands. In some cases, these systems are paired with functional electrical stimulation (FES), which delivers small electrical pulses to the affected muscles. This combination can further enhance motor relearning by providing both neural and muscular stimulation simultaneously. With growing scientific development and innovation, BCI assisted rehabilitation is gaining interest as a promising addition to standard therapy protocols. It offers the potential for faster recovery, improved patient engagement, and greater independence for individuals affected by neurological injuries. Complementing these approaches, bioelectronic medicine targets peripheral autonomic pathways such as the vagus nerve to treat inflammatory and autoimmune disorders. By modulating physiological responses through precisely timed electrical stimulation, bioelectronic interventions expand the therapeutic landscape and illustrate the broader potential of neural interfaces in rehabilitation.

### 8.1.3 Mental Disorders, Neurodegenerative Disease and Diagnosis

Mental disorders and neurodegenerative diseases are complex conditions that often present challenges in diagnosis, monitoring, and treatment. Although traditionally treated using clinical assessments and pharmaceutical interventions, BCI technologies are beginning to show promise in supplementing existing methods. These technologies offer the possibility of capturing brain activity in real time, providing insights that are often difficult to obtain through conventional approaches. While BCIs were originally developed for motor control applications, their use has expanded into the domain of cognitive and emotional disorders. For example, Parkinson's disease is a well-known neurodegenerative condition that primarily affects movement. It is caused by the gradual degeneration of dopamine producing neurons in the brain, leading to tremors, muscle rigidity, and bradykinesia. Although not a mental disorder, Parkinson's disease often includes cognitive and emotional symptoms. Invasive BCI approaches, such as deep brain stimulation, have been used to alleviate these motor symptoms by delivering targeted electrical stimulation to specific brain regions. These techniques have shown significant success in reducing tremors and improving motor control.

BCI technologies are also contributing to the early detection and diagnosis of various mental health and neurodegenerative conditions. Noninvasive techniques such as EEG allow researchers and clinicians to analyze brain activity and identify neural markers associated with specific disorders. These markers can serve as indicators of atypical brain function and provide valuable diagnostic information. Some important examples include the following:

- Mismatch negativity (MMN) responses have been found to differ in individuals with major depressive disorder [104], ADHD [105], and autism [106] spectrum conditions.
- Steady-state visually evoked potential (SSVEP) does not show habituation effect in individuals who suffer from migraine-related disorders [107].
- The default mode network (DMN), which is active during rest and internal thought, shows abnormal patterns in individuals with cognitive impairment and behavioral disorders [108].
- The P300 response, a positive deflection in brain signals following a stimulus, is often delayed or reduced in conditions such as schizophrenia [109], Alzheimer's disease [110], and attention-related disorders.
- Frontal alpha asymmetry, a measure of the difference in alpha wave activity between the brain's left and right frontal regions, has been associated with emotional regulation [111] and is often imbalanced in individuals with anxiety and depression.
- Gamma band activity, which supports perceptual and cognitive integration, is frequently diminished in individuals with schizophrenia [112] and autism [113].
- Event related desynchronization (ERD) during motor or cognitive tasks varies in individuals with Parkinson's disease [114] and mood disorders [115], offering insights into altered brain dynamics.
- Resting state connectivity, especially between the frontal and parietal lobes, shows disruptions in individuals with attention-related conditions and executive function impairments [116].

These examples represent only a subset of ongoing research into the diagnostic capabilities of BCI. Many current methods involve the use of ML algorithms to classify patterns in brain activity and distinguish between healthy and disordered states. Although still in development, these systems offer the possibility of creating reliable and objective diagnostic tools. As research continues, it is likely that BCI-based neuromarkers will play an increasingly important role in the early detection, monitoring, and personalized treatment of mental and neurodegenerative conditions.

### 8.1.4 Neurofeedback and Augmentation

Neurofeedback is a self-regulation technique in which individuals receive real-time information about their brain activity, typically measured through noninvasive methods such as EEG or functional near-infrared spectroscopy (fNIRS). By observing their own brainwave patterns, individuals can learn to consciously influence specific aspects of their neural activity. This process is often described as a form of brain training, where users are guided to modify activity in targeted brain regions to achieve specific cognitive or emotional outcomes. The foundation of neurofeedback lies in operant conditioning. Individuals are provided with auditory or visual cues that reflect changes in brain activity, and over time, they learn to adjust these signals voluntarily. For example, increasing alpha wave activity may lead to a calming effect, while enhancing beta activity might improve alertness and focus. These capabilities have made neurofeedback an increasingly popular approach in both clinical and nonclinical settings.

Neurofeedback has shown promising results in treating a variety of mental health-related conditions. Research has demonstrated its effectiveness in reducing symptoms of attention-deficit/hyperactivity disorder (ADHD), major depressive disorder, post-traumatic stress disorder (PTSD), and autism spectrum disorder (ASD). In individuals with autism, for instance, training focused on regulating theta [117] and alpha band [118] activity has been associated with improvements in social behavior, emotional control, and attention. Similarly, individuals with depression have been taught to strengthen activity in prefrontal regions associated with positive emotional processing [119], resulting in measurable improvements in mood and cognitive flexibility. The core aim of these BCI application is learning to recognize and control abnormal/normal patterns of brain activity and by doing so, individuals can induce more balanced and adaptive brain function. Neurofeedback approaches are independent of any external stimulation or pharmacological intervention and only rely on the brain's inherent capacity for self-regulation and neuroplasticity. This makes it an attractive option for those seeking noninvasive and personalized approaches to mental and cognitive health.

The concept of neurofeedback can be connected to broader idea known as neural augmentation. When individuals gain the ability to enhance their mental performance, emotional stability, or attentional control through training, their brain function may be considered augmented. This augmentation is not limited to correcting deficits but can also involve improving skills in healthy individuals. For example, neurofeedback has been used in high-performance settings such as sports [120], artistic performance, and military training to optimize focus [121], reduce stress, and enhance resilience. Whether used for therapeutic recovery or neural enhancement, it reflects the potential of BCIs to support individuals in achieving more effective control over their own mental states. As technologies continue to evolve and become more accessible, neurofeedback is likely to play a growing role in both clinical treatment and human augmentation.

## 8.2 Entertainment

Beyond its foundational role in clinical and assistive technologies, BCI technology has also begun to show applications for healthy individuals, particularly in the field of entertainment. This transition is perhaps not surprising, as many people are naturally intrigued by the idea of controlling digital environments using only their brain signals, aka thoughts. The concept of "mind-controlled" interaction has captured the public imagination, and BCI offers a path toward realizing this idea in practical ways. A notable example is the first human subject with paralysis below the shoulders implanted with Neuralink's N1 chip, who demonstrated the ability to play video games using brain signals alone [122]. In addition to regaining voluntary motor control through the implanted system, this individual was also able to interact with digital content without using traditional input devices. Such breakthroughs highlight the growing potential for BCI to offer immersive and engaging experiences beyond the medical domain.

However, the broader adoption of BCI in entertainment has so far been driven largely by noninvasive technologies. Consumer grade EEG headsets such as those offered by Emotiv, NeuroSky, and OpenBCI have made it feasible for developers and hobbyists to experiment with BCI-based control in gaming and multimedia applications. These headsets are affordable, portable, and relatively easy to use via provided tools, making them well suited for casual environments and personal use. As a result, BCI has entered the mainstream primarily through the lenses of gaming, personalization, and interactive media.

### 8.2.1 Gaming

Gaming is considered one of the most significant growing industries globally, and it has often served as a testing ground for new technologies as well. Many of the tools now central to augmented reality (AR), virtual reality (VR), and mixed reality (MR) originally gained traction through gaming platforms. In this sense, the gaming community has always been open to experimentation and innovation, and BCI naturally fits into this culture of technological exploration. Gamer continuously seek ways to enhance control, immersion, and performance. BCI introduces a novel form of interaction by enabling users to influence game environments using brain signals. This has led to an increasing interest in integrating BCI into both commercial and experimental game design. Developers and researchers have created brain-controlled interfaces for popular games such as Minecraft, Halo, and

Call of Duty, as well as entirely new games built from the ground up to respond to neural activity by commercial companies as well.

The types of BCI used in gaming often draw from multiple paradigms. For example, MI paradigms, which are traditionally used in motor function restoration and rehabilitation, have been adapted to simulate movement or control virtual avatars. Reactive paradigms such as SSVEP and rapid serial visual presentation (RSVP) allow users to make selections or issue commands by focusing on visual stimuli. In more complex systems, cognitive states such as attention, mental workload, and emotional engagement are also monitored and used as input variables. These approaches can be combined to produce a multi-layered control system that allows for richer and more dynamic interactions within the game world. In addition to modifying existing games, there is a growing category of applications that are designed entirely around BCI. These games aim not only to entertain but also to promote cognitive engagement, emotional regulation, and mental training. For instance, some games are designed to reward players for achieving a calm or focused mental state, helping users develop mindfulness, and self-regulation skills in a gamified environment. We have also discussed gamification elements in Chapter 7.

As BCI-related hardware continues to improve and signal processing becomes more sophisticated, the boundary between intention and action in virtual environments is expected to become increasingly seamless. While current systems still face limitations in terms of accuracy and responsiveness, the trajectory suggests a future where BCI becomes a common feature in gaming setups, offering new dimensions of personalization, challenge, and immersion.

#### 8.2.1.1 Games Designed with BCI

A growing number of games have been developed, which span a variety of genres and platforms, from casual desktop games to immersive VR. The following are notable examples of BCI specific games and systems:

- **NeuroRacer**: Developed by researchers at the University of California, San Francisco (UCSF), this neurofeedback-based game uses EEG and performance data to adapt its difficulty in real time. *NeuroRacer* trains and assesses cognitive abilities such as sustained attention, working memory, and multitasking, and has been shown to improve these functions in both younger and older adults [84].
- **NeuroSky and Emotiv Headset Games**: Consumer grade EEG devices such as those from NeuroSky and Emotiv have enabled users to play simple interactive games through mental commands or emotional states. These include games where players move objects, race cars, or perform tasks like lifting and pushing items using measured states such as attention, calmness, or meditation.

- **BCI-controlled Drones and Simulations**: Some BCI-integrated experiences involve controlling drones or navigating flight simulators through mental imagery or visual attention. These games often employ paradigms such as MI or SSVEP, allowing users to direct movement, adjust speed, or perform maneuvers by focusing on specific mental tasks or visual cues [123].
- **BrainArena**: A competitive multiplayer game in which players use EEG signals to control game actions based on cognitive states such as focus or engagement. Rather than using hand-based input, players must manage their attention levels to outperform opponents, promoting the development of sustained mental control and cognitive endurance [87].
- **VR Cognitive Games**: BCI enhanced VR applications dynamically adjust the game environment in response to real-time measures of mental workload, emotional arousal, or cognitive fatigue. These games create immersive and personalized experiences by unlocking content or altering game dynamics according to the player's internal mental state [124, 125].

These examples highlight the creative ways in which BCI is being applied within the gaming industry developed by BCI user or commercial companies.

#### 8.2.1.2 BCI on Mainstream Games

While many BCI applications are designed for dedicated experimental games, researchers and developers have also begun integrating BCI into well-known commercial titles. These efforts are often experimental, led by academic groups or open-source communities, but they demonstrate the growing interest in applying BCI to mainstream gaming environments. Such adaptations allow users to interact with complex, dynamic worlds using only their cognitive or emotional states. Below are several prominent examples:

- **Minecraft (Mojang) [126]**: Perhaps the most widely used mainstream game in BCI research, Minecraft's open-world sandbox nature and support for community modding have made it ideal for prototyping brain-controlled interaction. Various labs and developers have built plugins enabling control of actions such as block placement, movement, or object selection using motor imagery and visual focus paradigms. Minecraft is also attracted application in BCI training for children and in neurorehabilitation contexts.
- **Skyrim (Bethesda) [127]**: Community-driven projects have explored the use of cognitive states to control spell casting or dialogue choices in Skyrim. For instance, a relaxed mental state might trigger a healing spell, while heightened attention could activate combat abilities. These projects explore immersive storytelling augmented by neural feedback.

- **Counter-strike: Global Offensive (Valve) [128]**: Research groups have tested the use of BCI in fast reaction scenarios such as crouching, weapon switching, or issuing tactical commands. Although the precision required in competitive shooters presents challenges, these experiments provide insights into reaction time, fatigue, and decision-making under pressure.
- **Assassin's Creed (Ubisoft) [129]**: Demonstrations have explore Assassin's Creed style game on how real-time emotional states, such as stress or calmness detected via EEG, could affect gameplay. For example, combat mechanics or narrative pacing could adapt dynamically depending on the player's mental state, offering a more personalized and emotionally responsive gaming experience.
- **Valorant and League of Legends (Riot Games) [129]**: In exploratory setups, EEG signals have been used to monitor attention levels and mental fatigue during gameplay. While not used for direct in-game control, these signals offer strategic feedback that could influence team coordination and performance optimization. Such integrations hint at the potential of BCI in esports training and cognitive enhancement.

In all these cases, gaming is used not only for entertainment but also as a testing platform for complex signal interpretation, feedback systems, and real-time BCI interaction. Many of these games also help improve focus, reaction time, memory, and motor imagery, which makes them useful for training and neurorehabilitation. As the technology becomes more accessible, BCI in gaming is expected to play a major role in both the development and public acceptance of brain-based control systems.

### 8.2.2 Personalization

BCI-based personalization is an early stage but growing field with limited to no widely available application at the moment. BCI-based personalization is an approach that allows presented content such as entertainment material, educational modules, or digital book content to adapt in real time based on brain signals in a way that maximizes arousal and valence. Such applications aim to keep the user engaged by adjusting the experience based on their cognitive and emotional state. Such applications have mostly been tested in laboratory settings, particularly in relation to learning, where the difficulty level adapts to match the individual's cognitive load or attention level. Similar experiments have been carried out in gaming environments where game complexity, pace, or challenge changes depending on the player's current mental state and part of game mechanics, as discussed in Chapter 7.

## 8.3 Workplace

The application of BCI technology in the workplace is a topic of ongoing debate, marked by both excitement and concern. While the idea of using brain signals in professional environments may raise ethical and privacy-related questions, it also presents promising opportunities. These include enhancing employee productivity, supporting cognitive well-being, and optimizing task allocation based on individual mental states and capabilities. The common use of BCI in workplace settings aims to gain deeper insights into employees' cognitive and emotional states during task performance. This information can be used to improve learning outcomes, monitor mental workload, evaluate performance in real time, and even assist in making task assignments that align with a person's cognitive strengths. The ultimate goal is to create environments that are not only more efficient but also more responsive to the needs of employees.

One of the emerging directions in this space is the use of BCI for performance monitoring. This refers to the process of assessing brain activity while employees engage in work-related tasks in order to infer levels of attention, mental fatigue, stress, or cognitive load. With this data, organizations could, in theory, make informed decisions about when to intervene such as by offering a break, reallocating tasks, or providing support thereby maintaining optimal productivity while safeguarding employee well-being. Despite the conceptual promise, this field is still in its early stages, and real-world implementation remains limited. There are no widely adopted BCI systems used routinely in professional environments today. However, a few experimental and research-oriented initiatives provide insight into what such applications might look like in the future:

- **SAP Research Initiative**: In a collaboration between SAP and research institutions, an experimental setup was developed to explore how BCI could be used to monitor cognitive load during complex problem-solving tasks. The findings suggested that real-time brain data could help employees recognize when their attention was declining, thereby improving focus management and task efficiency in high cognitive demand environments such as software development [130].
- **Applications in Defense Settings**: Although military operations are distinct from conventional workplace settings, they often involve similar concerns about performance, fatigue, and decision-making under pressure. Experimental BCI systems have been used to monitor neural indicators of stress, attention, and mental workload during critical missions. These efforts demonstrate how BCI could eventually be adapted for broader workplace contexts, particularly in high-risk or high-stakes professions [131].

While these examples remain largely experimental, they underscore the future potential of BCI as a tool for real-time cognitive analytics in the workplace. The integration of BCI into professional life will require not only technological readiness but also robust frameworks for governance and accountability.

### 8.3.1 Learning and Performance

BCI technology has the potential to significantly enhance learning and task performance in workplace settings. By using noninvasive brain signals such as EEG and fNIRS, these systems can assess an individual's cognitive and emotional state in real time. Based on this assessment, the system can dynamically modify the structure, difficulty, or pacing of tasks to better align with the user's mental condition. This technique is often referred to as adaptive training or dynamic task arrangement. For example, when a system detects signs of mental fatigue or cognitive overload, it may suggest a brief rest period or shift the user to a less demanding activity. Conversely, when high levels of attention or engagement are identified, the system can increase task complexity to maintain cognitive stimulation. This form of responsiveness not only supports more efficient learning but also helps reduce the risk of burnout by respecting the learner's cognitive limits.

Such adaptive environments holds significant potential in improving both individual learning outcomes and overall workplace performance. They are especially promising in high-performance demanding environment, for example, air traffic controller (ATC). In aviation and emergency response training, for instance, BCI systems are being used experimentally to monitor the mental workload of trainee pilots in simulation [132] and ATC [133, 134]. When indicators of stress or mental fatigue are detected, the simulation environment can be adjusted in real time either by simplifying the task or by providing supportive feedback to ensure that the training remains effective without overloading the individual. Adaptive arrangement can be used to create a feedback-rich learning loop, where the training is not only tailored to the user's skill level but also continuously adapted to their current mental state. Over time, such systems may allow for more personalized and efficient professional development, improving both individual resilience and overall workforce capability.

### 8.3.2 Resilience

Another important application of BCI is in supporting cognitive well-being in workplace. In this context, BCI can be used not to monitor employees passively, but rather to inform them with tools for managing stress and mental workload. One of the key goals here is to help individuals develop cognitive resilience. Resilience refers to the capacity to recover from periods of intense cognitive demand or emotional stress and to return to a functional and balanced mental state. Chronic cognitive overload is a known contributor to reduced workplace productivity, burnout, and diminished quality of decision-making. BCI systems, particularly those based on neurofeedback, can offer a promising avenue for building resilience by training individuals to self-regulate their own brain activity.

Through repeated neurofeedback sessions, users learn to recognize the neural patterns associated with stress, anxiety, or mental fatigue and gradually develop strategies to modulate these patterns. This may involve increasing alpha wave activity to promote relaxation or decreasing theta or beta activity to improve focus and reduce anxiety. Over time, this form of cognitive self-regulation can improve emotional stability, attentional control, and resistance to cognitive fatigue. Although no large-scale BCI system for resilience training is currently in formal use within workplace environments, several related commercial solutions are available. These include wearable EEG-based wellness devices that offer neurofeedback for stress reduction and mindfulness training known as Muse.

## 8.4 Neural Interface Applications Beyond BCIs

While BCI application have central role in neural interface; however, there are many neural interface systems already play essential roles in clinical and therapeutic settings, providing sensory restoration, motor rehabilitation, and neuromodulation capabilities. These set of neural interface follow same principles of sensing, decoding, stimulation, and closed-loop control translate across systems. Let's look at some of these applications.

### 8.4.1 Cochlear Implants

Cochlear implants bypass damaged cochlear hair cells and directly stimulate the auditory nerve through an array of implanted electrodes that run along the cochlea [135]. Unlike conventional hearing aids, which amplify sound, cochlear implants convert acoustic signals into electrical patterns that encode frequency, amplitude, and temporal information. These patterns are delivered to the auditory nerve, allowing the brain to interpret them as sound. Modern systems include an external microphone, sound processor, and transmitter paired with an internal receiver-stimulator and electrode array. Advances in signal processing algorithms have dramatically improved speech comprehension, particularly in noisy environments. Bilateral cochlear implantation and hybrid electro-acoustic stimulation have further expanded the clinical population that can benefit. As one of the most successful neural prostheses, cochlear implants restore meaningful hearing to individuals with severe-to-profound hearing loss and continue to evolve through enhanced coding strategies, ML-based noise reduction, and fully implantable designs.

### 8.4.2 Retinal Implants

Retinal implants provide artificial vision to individuals with degenerative retinal diseases such as retinitis pigmentosa or age-related macular degeneration [136]. These disorders cause photoreceptor loss while leaving downstream retinal ganglion cells partially intact. Retinal prostheses such as the Argus II system substitute photoreceptor function by capturing visual scenes through an external camera mounted on glasses. The image is processed and wirelessly transmitted to an implanted microelectrode array positioned on the retinal surface (epiretinal) or beneath it (subretinal). Electrical stimulation of retinal ganglion cells elicits patterned visual percepts known as phosphenes. While current systems provide low-resolution vision, they enable basic tasks such as detecting motion, navigating high-contrast environments, or recognizing large objects. Ongoing research aims to improve pixel density, biocompatibility, power delivery, and naturalistic encoding of visual information, with next-generation systems exploring optogenetics, photovoltaic stimulation, and cortical-level visual prostheses.

### 8.4.3 Somatosensory Neuroprosthetics

Somatosensory neuroprosthetics seek to restore touch perception in individuals using robotic or prosthetic limbs by interfacing directly with the somatosensory nervous system [137]. These systems deliver tactile feedback by stimulating peripheral nerves, dorsal column pathways, or the somatosensory cortex to evoke controlled, naturalistic sensations. Techniques include intraneural microelectrode arrays, cuff electrodes, and electrocorticography (ECoG)-based stimulation. Psychophysical calibration allows the mapping of stimulation patterns to specific percepts such as pressure, vibration, temperature, or proprioception. Integrating sensory feedback into prosthetic control significantly improves dexterity, embodiment, and motor performance by closing the sensorimotor loop. Recent breakthroughs have demonstrated stable multi-year sensory restoration and high-resolution tactile perception, enabling users to grasp delicate objects, adjust grip force, and perform complex manipulation with reduced visual dependence. These advances represent a major step toward biomimetic prostheses capable of restoring near-natural sensation.

### 8.4.4 Peripheral Nerve Interfaces

Peripheral nerve interfaces enable bidirectional communication with the peripheral nervous system, allowing decoding of motor intent and delivery of sensory or therapeutic stimulation [138]. Current technologies include noninvasive surface electrodes, partially invasive cuff electrodes that wrap around nerves, and highly invasive intraneural electrodes such as longitudinal intrafascicular electrodes (LIFEs), transversal intrafascicular multichannel electrodes (TIMEs), and regenerative sieve electrodes. Electroneurography and electromyography signals recorded from these interfaces can decode fine motor commands for prosthetic control, while electrical stimulation can restore sensory feedback or modulate autonomic pathways. Peripheral interfaces are also used in bioelectronic medicine to regulate inflammatory responses via vagus nerve stimulation. Challenges remain in long-term stability, immune response, and electrode durability, but recent advances in flexible electronics, soft biointerfaces, and wireless implantable platforms continue to expand their clinical potential.

### 8.4.5 Spinal Cord Interfaces

Spinal cord interfaces target ascending and descending pathways to restore motor and sensory function after spinal cord injury [139]. Epidural electrical stimulation (EES) applies electrical pulses to the dorsal surface of the spinal cord, enabling individuals with severe paralysis to regain stepping, standing, and even voluntary limb movement. More invasive intraspinal microstimulation techniques place electrodes within spinal gray matter to activate specific motor pools with fine spatial precision. These interfaces exploit the intrinsic capabilities of spinal circuits to generate coordinated locomotor patterns when properly modulated. Combining EES with real-time decoding of motor intent from cortical or peripheral signals has yielded powerful closed-loop systems, allowing users to intentionally control their limbs. Furthermore, spinal interfaces show promise in neuropathic pain management and autonomic regulation. Continued integration of adaptive stimulation, machine learning, and personalized electrode configurations is rapidly advancing the field.

## 8.5 Summary

The evolving field of BCIs has moved far beyond its original clinical purpose, branching into applications across medicine, rehabilitation, entertainment, and the workplace. BCIs aim to provide a direct communication link between the brain and external devices, which is an innovation capable of reshaping how humans interact with technology and the world. Medical applications remain the most advanced, with BCIs restoring motor functions, supporting rehabilitation, assisting in mental health assessment, and enabling neurofeedback-based interventions. At the same time, BCIs are gaining popularity among healthy users, particularly in gaming and immersive experiences, where they provide new levels of engagement, personalization, and cognitive exploration. In professional contexts, BCIs offer opportunities for adaptive learning, performance monitoring, safety enhancement, and cognitive resilience building, though they also raise important ethical considerations related to privacy, autonomy, fairness, and responsible implementation.

Although BCIs are the most visible and widely explored form of neural interface, they belong to a much broader ecosystem of technologies, including neuromodulation systems, peripheral nerve interfaces, sensory prostheses, and bioelectronic medicine. These complementary systems highlight the wider landscape in which BCIs operate and reinforce the idea that neural interfaces as a whole are poised to transform how people work, learn, play, and heal.

# 9

# Enhancing Human Capabilities with Neural Interfaces

We explored the broad benefits of brain–computer interfaces (BCIs) in Chapter 8, spanning applications from clinical treatments to entertainment for healthy individuals. In recent years, there has been a notable increase in interest and investment from private companies in BCI. Among the leading contributors in invasive BCI development are *Neuralink*, *Paradromics*, and *Synchron*. In the non-invasive space, companies such as *Muse*, *Emotiv*, *Mendi*, and *Meta* are actively advancing technologies, particularly those based on electroencephalography (EEG) and functional near-infrared spectroscopy (fNIRS). These private sector efforts have significantly boosted confidence in the potential of BCI technologies. It is not wrong to call it significant hype; however, a positive encouragement as well for greater participation from both the research community and the general public. As a result, there is a growing interest in restoring lost human functions with BCI, including speech, vision, and motor control. This domain is often informally referred to as "thought reading BCI," encompassing efforts to decode inner speech, visual experiences, and other cognitive processes. The concept remains closely aligned with the original vision of BCI technology, which aims to interpret human thoughts directly and accurately and eventually to augment them. Although the full potential of such systems has not yet been realized, the pace of progress in both BCI and artificial intelligence (AI) suggests we are approaching a new era of technologies. This chapter explores emerging BCI research aimed at improving, enhancing, and extending human capabilities, positioning these BCI systems as a new class of human enhancement technologies.

## 9.1 Speech and Mental Imagery in BCI

Human thoughts arise from a complex integration of multiple cognitive processes, shaped by memory, emotion, and sensory inputs such as vision, sound, smell, and touch, as well as by accumulated experiences. Within the current landscape of BCI research, these mental processes are often categorized into two primary areas of interest: speech and mental imagery. Both are fundamental components of human cognition. These two domains are particularly compelling to researchers, perhaps because much of our daily thinking involves internal dialogue and mental visualization. Such inner experiences play a critical role in information processing, problem-solving, and decision-making [140]. Consider, for instance, the potential of a BCI capable of translating inner speech directly into digital text or projecting mental images onto a screen to communicate ideas, memories, or creative concepts. These capabilities could not only enhance everyday interaction but also have profound implications for accessibility and for extending human cognitive abilities. A BCI that decodes imagined speech could enable individuals who are mute to communicate solely through thought. Likewise, decoding mental imagery could offer novel applications for introspection or even clinical diagnosis. In the field of mental health, the ability to interpret mental imagery may provide new tools for understanding and treating conditions such as schizophrenia or post-traumatic stress disorder (PTSD).

Although BCI technology remains in its early stages and is not yet capable of fully realizing these possibilities, research and development are advancing rapidly. The following sections explore the domains of speech and mental imagery in detail, examining both the current state of the art and the emerging applications of BCI in the context of human enhancement.

### 9.1.1 Mental Speech BCI

Mental speech BCI aim to decode internal or unspoken verbal thoughts directly from brain activity, bypassing the need for vocal cords or muscular articulation. This technology is often referred to as a speech prosthesis, primarily aim to develop for individuals who have lost the ability to speak due to conditions such as paralysis, aphonia, or neurological disorders like amyotrophic lateral sclerosis (ALS) or stroke. Recent advances [141–143], particularly in invasive BCI systems, have demonstrated promising results. Using high-resolution neural recordings, researchers have successfully reconstructed silent or imagined speech with accuracies ranging from 60 to 70%. These breakthroughs mark a significant step toward restoring communication for individuals with severe speech impairments. Non-invasive approaches, though currently limited in spatial resolution and accuracy but still able to achieve around 30% accuracy and showing promising results. The use of generative AI in these BCI systems, especially large language model (LLM), has been instrumental in improving output quality by predicting and completing phrases based on partial neural data.

Mental speech BCIs are grounded in our understanding of the neural architecture of language. Key brain regions involved include Broca's area, associated with speech production; Wernicke's area, linked to language comprehension; and the supplementary motor area, which plays a role in speech planning and initiation. Invasive methods such as electrocorticography (ECoG) offer high temporal and spatial resolution, enabling the detection of fine-grained neural patterns associated with phonemes, syllables, and even entire words. These signals are then decoded using advanced machine learning (ML) algorithms to reconstruct the user's intended speech. Noninvasive modalities, including EEG and fNIRS face greater challenges due to signal attenuation, lower spatial resolution, and susceptibility to noise. However, these limitations are partially offset by the safety, accessibility, and scalability of such acquisition methods, therefore making them more feasible for widespread use. There are attempts to create hybrid systems that combine multiple noninvasive signals to augment neural data with contextual cues from AI models to bridge the performance gap between invasive and noninvasive techniques. Although mental speech BCIs are still evolving, their potential applications extend far beyond medical rehabilitation. These technologies hold promise for augmenting everyday cognitive functions and enabling new forms of interaction.

Some potential speculative applications that highlight the enhancement of human capabilities with the help of mental speech BCI could be:

- **Thought-to-text Interfaces (TTUIs)**: Future BCIs may enable users to compose written content such as emails, documents, or software code solely through internal speech. By reducing dependence on physical input devices, such interfaces could significantly enhance efficiency and productivity, particularly in cognitively demanding or hands-busy environments.
- **Brain-to-brain Interfaces for Silent Communication**: Mental speech decoding could facilitate silent, speechless communication by transmitting internally generated verbal content directly to another individual or computational system. This capability would be advantageous in contexts where spoken communication is impractical or undesirable. Although the prospect of direct brain-to-brain communication remains highly speculative, it continues to attract sustained interest in neuroscience, cognitive science, and human–machine interface research.
- **Thought-to-AI Interaction**: Advanced BCIs may eventually support seamless interaction with AI agents capable of interpreting internal commands. Such systems could operate as real-time cognitive assistants or even as "Copilot" [144] BCIs by supporting memory recall, conducting on-demand information retrieval, and assisting with complex decision-making processes. In this capacity, thought-to-AI interfaces would function as a form of cognitive extension or augmentation, integrating AI directly into the user's internal deliberative processes.
- **Multilingual Communication**: BCIs capable of decoding imagined speech may also enable real-time translation from one language to another. This

would allow users to communicate across linguistic boundaries without the need for deliberate language switching or manual translation, potentially transforming multilingual interaction in both personal and professional settings.

- **Creative Expression and Ideation**: By externalizing unspoken or abstract internal speech, mental speech BCIs could facilitate novel forms of creative expression. Artists, writers, and designers may be able to rapidly convert conceptual ideas into tangible digital forms, thereby accelerating ideation processes and reducing barriers between internal cognition and external creation.

### 9.1.2 Mental Imagery BCI

Mental imagery refers to the cognitive process of visualizing scenes, objects, or abstract concepts in the absence of direct sensory input. It is a fundamental function of the human mind, allowing individuals to simulate experiences, rehearse actions, and conceptualize ideas without interacting with the physical world. This internal visualization process plays a vital role in memory recall, imagination, planning, emotional regulation, and even motor preparation. Numerous studies [145, 146] suggest that individuals who can vividly generate mental imagery often perform better in problem-solving tasks, spatial reasoning challenges, and creative pursuits. Dreams themselves may be understood as a spontaneous and often vivid form of mental imagery. Occurring primarily during rapid eye moment (REM) sleep, they typically consist of rich visual scenes, emotionally charged content, and internally generated narratives or dialogues. This spontaneous simulation of sensory and cognitive content further underscores the brain's capacity to construct immersive, image-based experiences from within.

BCI research of mental imagery seek to decode and reconstruct these internally generated visual experiences directly from neural activity. This emerging class of systems can be referred to as visual prostheses. The ultimate objective is to create interfaces capable of translating mental imagery into visual representations in real time, thereby unlocking new modes of communication, expression, and introspection. Imagine, for instance, a future where individuals could sketch by simply visualizing an image or convey deeply personal memories to a therapist through a visual playback of their mental imagery. Such capabilities would not only enhance creativity and therapeutic practices but also provide a bridge between subjective experience and objective expression.

Much of the early progress in this field has been achieved using functional magnetic resonance imaging (fMRI). fMRI enables researchers to identify and decode patterns of neural activity in visual cortical regions, particularly those responsible for low-level visual processing such as color, orientation, and spatial layout [147, 148]. These works have demonstrated the ability to reconstruct simple visual stimuli including shapes, letters, and scenes with increasing fidelity based on these patterns. Although fMRI provides high spatial resolution, it is limited by its size and lack of portability. For broader accessibility, researchers have begun exploring noninvasive methods such as EEG, fNIRS as well as MEG. While these approaches face limitations in signal spatial resolution, ongoing advancements in signal processing and ML are making it increasingly feasible to decode mental imagery from such modalities. While still in the experimental phase, the potential applications of mental imagery BCIs for human enhancement are both broad and profound. Future developments may enable entirely new forms of expression, perception, and interaction. Some speculative yet promising directions include:

- **Mental Imagery Communication**: In the future, individuals may be able to share visual thoughts or memories directly with others through mental imagery BCIs. Such systems could allow one person's internal visual experience to be decoded and rendered for another, creating a new modality of interpersonal communication that bypasses language entirely. This might open up new forms of empathy, storytelling, or even collaborative visualization for design or education.
- **Therapeutic Visualization Tools**: Mental imagery BCIs could provide clinicians with access to reconstructed visualizations of a patient's internal experiences. Though speculative, such tools might aid in the diagnosis and treatment of psychological conditions like PTSD, anxiety, or phobias by allowing therapists to view or analyze distressing mental images as they are internally generated. This could offer new dimensions for exposure therapy, cognitive restructuring, or emotional regulation.
- **Creative Visualization**: Future creative professionals may be able to externalize their imagined scenes, objects, or artistic concepts directly from mental imagery, without traditional sketching, modeling, or design tools. Such capabilities could streamline early ideation, accelerate prototyping, and reduce barriers between abstract thought and concrete creation. Artists, designers, and filmmakers might use these systems to capture fleeting visions that would otherwise be difficult to articulate.
- **Dream Recording**: With further advancements, it may become possible to decode and reconstruct dream imagery in near real-time. This could enable the recording and playback of dreams for personal reflection or psychological study. While this remains highly speculative, such a tool could offer researchers unprecedented access to the subconscious mind, potentially enriching the understanding of memory consolidation, emotional processing, and symbolic cognition during sleep.

- **Mental Simulation and Problem-solving**: Mental imagery BCIs could serve as cognitive augmentation tools, allowing users to simulate hypothetical scenarios, visualize abstract problems, or mentally rehearse complex tasks. For example, a user might be able to visualize architectural spaces before they are built or mentally simulate the outcome of strategic decisions. Such applications, while still in the realm of speculation, could extend human cognition and decision-making in unprecedented ways.

## 9.2 Neuroadaptive BCI

The concept of a Neuroadaptive BCI refers to systems that continuously monitor, interpret, and respond to the user's cognitive and emotional states in real time. Traditional BCIs focus primarily on decoding explicit intentional commands such as imagined movement or internal speech, neuroadaptive BCIs emphasize the interpretation of implicit neural processes including attention, workload, fatigue, engagement, and affect. By adapting system behavior based on these internal states, neuroadaptive BCIs aim to optimize human–machine interaction, reduce cognitive load, and support more efficient task performance. This emerging paradigm shifts BCIs from only communication tools toward collaborative, context-sensitive system capable of dynamically regulating the interaction according to the user's fluctuating cognitive demands. Technically, neuroadaptive BCIs build upon advances in passive BCI, cognitive state monitoring, and adaptive human–computer interaction. These systems typically employ noninvasive modalities such as EEG or fNIRS, often in combination with other physiological signals including heart rate variability (HRV), electrodermal activity (EDA), or eye tracking. ML models are used to infer cognitive states from these multimodal signals and adjust system parameters accordingly. Such adjustments may involve modifying task difficulty, interface complexity, automation level, or feedback timing to maintain optimal user performance and engagement.

### 9.2.1 Key Characteristics

Neuroadaptive BCIs are still a growing fields; however, some of key characteristics of such system compared to traditional BCI systems are as follows:

- **Continuous Cognitive Monitoring**: Neuroadaptive BCIs continuously assess neural activity associated with cognitive workload, attentional fluctuations, fatigue, cognitive conflict, and affective states. By integrating these signals in real time, such systems can enable continuous estimate of the user's cognitive readiness and performance capacity.

- **Closed-loop Adaptation**: These systems employ closed-loop control in which decoded cognitive states drive dynamic adjustments to system parameters such as task difficulty, automation level, or feedback timing. Subsequent neural responses to these adaptations are monitored to refine the loop, enabling stable and context-sensitive interaction.
- **Hyperpersonalization Over Time**: Through sustained interaction, learning algorithms identify user-specific neural markers, behavioral patterns, and contextual factors. This enables progressively finer-grained personalization, allowing the BCI to anticipate cognitive demands and optimize support based on the individual's evolving cognitive profile and long-term adaptation patterns.
- **Implicit Interaction**: Existing BCIs rely on intentional commands or task-specific mental strategies, neuroadaptive BCIs may able to operate largely implicitly. They extract meaningful information from spontaneous neural activity, reducing the need for deliberate user effort and thereby promoting more naturalistic, low-burden interaction.

### 9.2.2 Examples and Current Progress Toward Neuroadaptive BCI

Recent research has demonstrated the feasibility of neuroadaptive principles across a wide range of application domains [149, 150]. For instance, systems capable of detecting lapses in attention or elevated workload have been integrated into aviation and driving simulators to adjust automation levels during periods of cognitive overload. In educational settings, cognitive state monitoring has been used to adapt instructional content based on neural indicators of engagement or confusion, thereby supporting individualized learning trajectories. Similarly, rehabilitation and neurofeedback environments have employed adaptive feedback mechanisms to maintain motivation, regulate task difficulty, and facilitate personalized therapeutic progress.

Neuroadaptive approaches have also shows better human-agent teaming, where agent could be physical human–robot collaboration (pHRC) [151]. These BCIs have demonstrated that real-time estimates of user workload, stress, or cognitive conflict to modulate robotic assistance levels during collaborative tasks. For example, a neuroadaptive robotic system may increase its physical support during periods of user fatigue or uncertainty or reduce its assistance when neural indicators suggest high confidence or sufficient motor capability. Such adaptive modulation enhances safety, efficiency, and user trust in pHRI scenarios while reducing cognitive and physical strain.

While this chapter has focused on individual enhancement, early research also suggests that BCIs could support group-level cognition and shared decision-making. These speculative multi-brain interfaces are discussed further in Chapter 12.

## 9.3 Natural BCI

The concept of a Natural BCI is an emerging and evolving notion within the broader field of BCI. Unlike well-defined paradigms in traditional BCI research such as MI or P300 speller systems, Natural BCI currently lacks a universally accepted definition. Rather, it represents a design philosophy and a research trajectory focused on creating systems that align more closely with the brain's spontaneous and intuitive modes of operation. As such, the term "Natural BCI" remains open to interpretation, yet its core aspiration is clear that facilitate brain-device interaction that feels as seamless and instinctive as ordinary human thought, perception, or action. Traditional BCIs often require users to perform cognitively demanding or artificial tasks, such as imagining specific movements or selecting symbols through focused attention. These methods, while effective in controlled settings, are typically slow, effortful, and cognitively taxing. In contrast, Natural BCIs aim to minimize or eliminate the need for such adaptation. Instead of training the brain to communicate with a machine, Natural BCIs focus on decoding naturally occurring mental states such as intentions, emotions, visual imagery, and internal speech in real time, and with minimal user effort.

In this vision, the interface becomes invisible where users interact with technology through their cognitive processes, as naturally as they would speak, reach, or decide. A Natural BCI ideally interprets brain activity passively or with little conscious effort, integrating smoothly into everyday environments. It adapts to the user rather than requiring the user to adapt to it. Achieving this level of fluidity requires a convergence of several disciplines, including neuroscience, AI, ML, and human-computer interaction. There is also need for models capable of understanding context, learning from sparse or noisy data, and personalizing interaction over time. Deep learning (DL) and transformer-based architectures, in particular, have shown promise in interpreting complex brain activity with greater nuance and adaptability.

### 9.3.1 Philosophy Behind Natural BCI

The human brain did not evolve to control cursors or robotic limbs, but it evolved for walking, talking, sensing, and interacting in a rich and dynamic environment. A natural BCI should therefore not demand the user to "think in code" or perform arbitrary mental tasks (such as imagining hand movement to move a cursor). Instead, it should tap into naturally occurring neural patterns associated with thought, intention, speech, perception, and emotion. The ultimate goal is to build a system where the user is not consciously aware of operating a BCI. It just becomes an extension of themselves. This idea aligns with how we currently use tools like smartphones or computers: the more intuitive the interface, the more "invisible" it becomes.

### 9.3.2 Key Components of a Natural BCI

Achieving this level of seamless integration requires more than high-accuracy decoding and a multidimensional system that adapts dynamically to both the user and their environment. The following are foundational components that characterize the emerging vision of Natural BCIs:

- **Adaptive Learning**: A Natural BCI must continually learn from and adapt to the unique neural patterns of each user. ML algorithms, especially those capable of incremental or online learning, enable the system to refine its decoding accuracy over time while accommodating neural variability due to fatigue, mood, or attention shifts.
- **Context Awareness**: Effective interpretation of brain signals depends on understanding the broader context in which those signals arise. This includes not only environmental factors, for example, whether the user is walking or reading but also internal states such as emotional tone, cognitive load, or social intent. By incorporating contextual awareness, the BCI can better infer user goals and reduce ambiguity.
- **Low Latency**: For the interface to feel truly natural, feedback and system responses must be nearly instantaneous. High latency introduces a perceptual disconnect between intention and action, which can disrupt the feeling of agency. Fast processing pipelines and optimized decoding models are essential for maintaining real-time interaction.
- **Minimal Training**: A natural interaction is low cognitive overhead. Users should be able to use the system with little to no explicit training. Ideally, a Natural BCI should work "out of the box" or improve rapidly through passive calibration and usage, not require users to learn mental strategies that diverge from their natural thought patterns.
- **Bidirectional Communication**: While most current BCIs focus on reading signals from the brain, a fully natural interface would also include feedback channels such as visual, auditory, or haptic feedback to close the sensorimotor loop. This bidirectional flow mirrors how humans naturally interact with the environment and is essential for developing systems that feel responsive, intuitive, and embodied.

### 9.3.3 Examples and Current Progress toward Natural BCI

Modern applications are moving toward natural interaction, even if still in their early stages. Some promising areas include:

- **Motor Intention Decoding**: Systems capable of detecting a user's intended limb movements from neural activity are becoming increasingly sophisticated. These interfaces allow individuals particularly those with motor impairments to control prosthetic limbs or robotic devices in real time, simply by intending to move. While many systems still rely on invasive implants, noninvasive approaches are also showing promise in translating natural motor planning into control signals.
- **Emotion-based Interaction**: BCIs that infer affective states such as stress, engagement, or relaxation are being explored in applications ranging from mental wellness to adaptive gaming. By detecting emotional responses in real time, these systems can tailor experiences to match the user's internal state, creating more personalized and supportive environments.
- **Smart Environment Control**: Natural BCIs are beginning to be integrated into smart home systems, allowing users to influence lighting, temperature, or media playback through subtle thought patterns or emotional cues. These systems aim to detect and respond to intention or affect without requiring deliberate command-based interaction.
- **Context Aware Decoding**: By combining brain activity with user behavior, location, or environmental conditions, BCIs can infer intent more accurately and naturally. This allows for proactive system responses that align with inferred goals, without requiring the user to issue explicit instructions.
- **Passive BCIs**: These systems continuously and unobtrusively monitor brain activity to detect changes in cognitive or emotional states. Unlike active BCIs, which require users to engage in specific mental tasks, passive BCIs gather insights in the background and are increasingly being used in fields like cognitive monitoring, workload, fatigue detection, and neurofeedback-based training.
- **Multimodal Integration**: Combining brain signals with other natural inputs such as eye tracking, facial expressions, or speech patterns enhances system robustness and interpretability. This multimodal approach reduces reliance on any single input channel and more closely mirrors the way humans communicate and perceive the world.
- **Zero-training Interfaces**: Emerging systems are exploring ways to eliminate lengthy user-specific training or calibration. By leveraging large scale ML models and transfer learning techniques, these BCIs can personalize decoding dynamically, making the interface immediately usable and adaptive over time.

- **Emotionally Intelligent Systems**: By interpreting subtle changes in mood or arousal, BCIs could eventually enable emotionally responsive applications in domains such as education, therapy, and entertainment. These systems might adapt their behavior to support motivation, engagement, or emotional well-being based on real-time affective feedback.

Together with progress in mental speech and imagery, represent early steps toward the realization of natural BCIs. While each presents technical and theoretical challenges, they collectively define a direction in which BCI is not only possible but transformative.

## 9.4 Multimodality and Multitasking in BCI

Most existing BCI systems are designed with a narrow operational focus, for example, rely on a single type of brain signals and are optimized for one specific task or command structure. While this approach has led to important breakthroughs in assistive communication, motor control, and neurofeedback, it imposes a fundamental limitation on the scope of interaction. Human cognition, in contrast, is inherently multimodal and multitasking. We process visual, auditory, emotional, and bodily information simultaneously while managing multiple goals and behaviors in parallel. A next-generation vision of BCI moves beyond single stream control by embracing multimodal and multitasking architectures. In such systems, multiple brain signal sources could combine invasive and noninvasive recordings with additional physiological data streams such as ECG, HRV, PPG, electrodermal activity (EDA), and others. These signals reflect various dimensions of cognitive and affective state, allowing for richer, more context-aware interpretation of user intent and condition.

In a multimodal, multitasking BCI system, users could potentially control several functions or devices concurrently. Consider, for example, a user operating a drone with MI while simultaneously adjusting its camera angle using internal speech. Or a physically impaired individual who manipulates a robotic arm through thought while interacting with a virtual interface via gaze or facial expression. Even for healthy users, such systems could offer cognitive or physical augmentation, enabling more efficient task execution in domains such as manufacturing, aviation, or military operations. Another scenario could involve dual pathways of control using overt physical movement for one task (e.g., typing or manipulating objects) and covert neural signals for another (e.g., controlling an exoskeleton or AR/VR system). In such contexts, cognitive load management becomes a central design challenge, as the system must continuously monitor and adapt to the user's attention, fatigue, and emotional state.

## 9.5 Summary

The field of BCI is rapidly evolving from a niche research domain into a transformative technology with the potential to significantly enhance human capabilities. As explored in this chapter, BCIs are no longer limited to clinical rehabilitation or assistive communication; they are beginning to redefine how we express thoughts, visualize ideas, and interact with machines. The growing momentum in both invasive and noninvasive BCI research driven by advances in neuroscience, AI, and private sector investment, has led to the development of applications that blur the boundary between mind and machine. Central to this progress are two emerging frontiers: mental speech and mental imagery decoding. These approaches offer the possibility of translating internal experiences such as silent speech or mental visual imagery into actionable outputs, enabling powerful new tools for communication, creativity, therapy, and cognition.

Mental speech BCIs aim to restore or augment verbal expression, especially for those who have lost the ability to speak, while also creating new pathways for hands-free, silent communication with devices or other individuals. Meanwhile, mental imagery BCIs promise to externalize inner visualizations, making it possible to share ideas, recall memories, or diagnose mental health conditions by decoding what the mind sees. Complementing these developments is the vision of a Natural BCI. An interface that operates as seamlessly and intuitively as a natural limb or spoken language. These systems emphasize low training, context sensitivity, and real-time adaptation to the user's mental state. They represent a philosophical and technological shift toward interfaces that feel like true extensions of the human mind.

Finally, the integration of multimodal and multitasking capabilities into BCIs suggests a future where brain signals work in harmony with other physiological inputs and external controls. This opens the door to sophisticated, parallel interactions supporting new forms of multitasking, adaptive environments, and even enhanced human-machine symbiosis. Together, these advances mark a new era of brain-interface technologies that move beyond restoration toward augmentation. They challenge conventional notions of communication, creativity, and consciousness, offering unprecedented ways to expand human potential. While many of these capabilities are still in early stages, the foundation is being laid for a future where thought itself becomes a primary interface.

As we move forward, continued cross-disciplinary collaboration will be essential linking neuroscience, engineering, ethics, and design to ensure that BCIs remain human-centered, equitable, and responsibly deployed. The dream of using thought to enhance action, expression, and understanding is no longer a distant vision. It is a rapidly approaching reality.

# 10

# Neuroethics

Neuroethics can be defined as field of ethics in neuroscience that examines the ethical, legal, and social implications of neuroscience. In this ever-growing field of neuroscience-based application, aka brain–computer interface (BCI) technologies, neuroethics became a highly important field to consider. The reason behind this is a more and more transition of BCI from experimental prototypes in research laboratories to practical tools in clinical, commercial, and even consumer settings. Therefore, ethical challenges surrounding their development and deployment grow ever more pressing. These BCI technologies promise to revolutionize the human experience by offering the ability to enable lost functions such as speech and mobility, and even enhance cognitive capacities such as attention and decision-making. In doing so, BCIs are redefining the boundaries between biology and technology, mind and machine. This unique relationship gives rise to a host of complex ethical issues, including risks of infringing on mental privacy, manipulation of thought and behavior, loss of autonomy, and widening social inequalities. As innovation accelerates and private industries become increasingly involved, questions of consent, data governance, safety, equity, and long-term impact move from theoretical to urgent. This chapter explores these ethical dimensions and their implications for individuals and society.

## 10.1 Responsible Technology Development

The ethical responsibility in developing BCI systems lies with scientists, engineers, industry leaders, clinicians, ethicists, and policymakers. These stakeholders are working collaboratively to ensure that BCI technologies are developed with a strong commitment to human well-being, dignity, and safety. Technology developers are required to weigh the benefits of innovation against potential harms for individuals and society. Invasive BCI systems, in particular, present unique physical and psychological risks. Responsible development therefore requires attention to both short-term effects and long-term implications. Table 10.1 summarizes the key principles for responsible BCI technology development.

**Table 10.1** Key principles of responsible BCI technology development.

| Ethical principle | Focus area | Key considerations | Recommended actions |
|---|---|---|---|
| **Informed and Inclusive Participation** | Consent and user autonomy | Clear communication of risks, benefits, alternatives; complexity in vulnerable populations | Implement dynamic consent processes; involve multidisciplinary oversight; ensure right to withdraw |
| **Vulnerability and Proxy Consent** | Ethical inclusion of at risk users | Children, nonverbal users, or cognitively impaired individuals may need proxy decision makers | Develop robust policy frameworks; clarify roles and limits of guardians or legal representatives |
| **Ongoing Consent Mechanisms** | Changes over time in BCI systems | Software updates, user adaptation, or risk shifts may alter the user experience | Re-consent protocols, regular user engagement, and transparent communication of changes |
| **Safety and Risk Mitigation** | Avoidance of harm during development and deployment | Invasive BCIs can cause physical, psychological, or long-term neurological harm | Prioritize rigorous preclinical and clinical testing; align development with evolving safety standards |
| **Equity and Accessibility** | Social inclusion and fairness | High-cost or institution-specific BCIs may worsen existing digital and health divides | Design affordable and usable solutions across diverse socioeconomic and geographic contexts |
| **Transparency and Accountability** | Trust building and independent validation | Conflicts of interest, closed research, or lack of community dialogue can erode public trust | Disclose financial ties; share methodologies and data; engage communities throughout development |

| Ethical principle | Focus area | Key considerations | Recommended actions |
|---|---|---|---|
| **Inclusive Design and Representation** | Reflecting diverse user needs in system design | Systems may not suit or benefit underrepresented populations | Co-design with diverse stakeholders; test inclusivity across demographics, languages, and abilities |
| **Public Trust and Ethical Governance** | Long-term sustainability and legitimacy of the field | Perceptions of manipulation, surveillance, or misuse may hinder societal adoption | Foster open communication, independent oversight, and enforceable ethical standards |

### 10.1.1 Ensuring Informed and Inclusive Participation

A central tenet of responsible technology development is the assurance of informed, voluntary, and inclusive participation from all individuals involved in the use or testing of BCI systems. Obtaining informed consent requires transparent and comprehensive communication of risks, benefits, alternatives, and uncertainties. This process becomes especially complex when involving vulnerable populations, such as children or individuals with cognitive impairments, requiring careful oversight and clear policy frameworks.

Informed consent must also be an ongoing process, particularly for long-term or adaptive BCI use, where system updates or changes in neural integration can alter user experiences. Mechanisms for re-consent, regular updates, and easy withdrawal are essential to protect autonomy throughout the user's engagement with the technology.

### 10.1.2 Neuroethics of Pediatric BCI Use

The use of BCI technologies in children raises distinct ethical challenges because developing brains are highly plastic, vulnerable, and shaped by long-term environmental and technological influences. Children often cannot provide fully informed consent, and their ability to understand risks, future implications, or changes in self-perception is limited. As a result, decisions about BCI participation typically fall to parents or legal guardians, whose assessments may not always align with the child's long-term interests or emerging autonomy. BCIs intended for pediatric populations whether for communication support, treatment of neurological conditions, or potential cognitive enhancement must therefore be approached with particular caution. Neurodevelopmental impacts, personality shifts, or changes in emotional regulation may be amplified in children compared to adults. Long-term effects are difficult to predict, especially when devices adapt over time through machine learning (ML) processes. This uncertainty requires conservative risk-benefit assessments and extended monitoring of developmental, cognitive, and emotional outcomes.

Ethical practice in pediatric BCI research and deployment should ensure that children are involved in decision-making to the extent possible, respecting their growing autonomy. Assent processes must be age-appropriate, transparent, and supportive. Withdrawal from BCI use should remain a protected right as a child matures, particularly if earlier decisions were made on their behalf. Safeguards must also address fairness and social pressures: children should not be subjected to BCI interventions for competitive academic or behavioral purposes, nor exposed to coercive expectations from institutions or caregivers.

Ultimately, neuroethics of pediatric BCI use emphasizes protection, developmental sensitivity, and respect for emerging autonomy of developing brain. BCI technologies for children should prioritize therapeutic necessity, minimize risk, and preserve the child's future ability to shape their own identity, agency, and life choices.

### 10.1.3 Balancing Innovation with Safety and Equity

Rapid advancements in artificial intelligence (AI), neural decoding, and hardware miniaturization bring new opportunities but also introduce uncertainties. Responsible innovation requires robust testing, long-term safety research, and regulatory standards that evolve with technological progress. Premature commercial deployment risks physical harm and undermines public trust.

Equity must also be prioritized. Without intentional design for accessibility, BCI technologies risk deepening existing social and economic divides by primarily benefiting privileged groups. Inclusive design, affordability strategies, and engagement with diverse communities from early stages are essential to ensure fair distribution of benefits.

## 10.2 Public and Social Perception of BCI Technology

The public and social perception of BCI technology refers to the collective attitudes, beliefs, expectations, and concerns held by individuals and communities regarding the development and use of BCIs. These perceptions are shaped by cultural values, media narratives, lived experiences, and historical trust in science. While many view BCIs as empowering tools for communication and mobility, others express anxiety about mind reading, surveillance, or loss of control. These concerns are heightened as BCIs move beyond clinical settings into consumer and commercial domains.

### 10.2.1 Cultural Dimensions of Public Acceptance

Cultural and spiritual frameworks influence how communities interpret the augmentation of brain function through technological means. Technologies such as cochlear implants have historically raised concerns about cultural identity, and similar tensions may emerge around BCIs [152]. Religious or metaphysical beliefs may also shape how communities perceive brain intervention, underscoring the importance of culturally sensitive design and engagement.

## 10.3 Identity, Agency, and Personhood

BCIs raise important questions about how technology interacts with human identity, agency, and personhood. Because they operate directly on neural activity, BCIs may alter how users perceive themselves, how they act, and how they relate to their own thoughts.

### 10.3.1 BCIs and the Sense of Self

Identity is shaped through bodily experience, emotion, memory, and social interaction. BCIs that restore or augment function may strengthen independence but can also introduce shifts in mood or cognition that feel unfamiliar. Adaptive BCIs that learn from users may subtly influence emotional states or preferences, raising questions about the boundaries of self-directed identity.

### 10.3.2 Agency and Control

Agency refers to the capacity to initiate and direct actions. BCIs complicate this because outputs arise from an interaction between human neural signals and algorithmic interpretation. Autocorrection, prediction, or misalignment between intention and execution may blur distinctions between voluntary and involuntary action, with implications for medical, social, and legal accountability.

### 10.3.3 Personhood and Ethical Considerations

When external systems become integrated into cognitive processes, distinctions between the user and the device may blur. Enhancement-oriented BCIs raise questions about fairness, social identity, and continuity of personhood. Safeguarding these dimensions is essential for ensuring BCIs enhance capability without compromising dignity or autonomy.

## 10.4 Mental Privacy and Cognitive Liberty

As BCIs gain the ability to decode intentions, emotions, and internal states, mental privacy becomes a central ethical concern. Mental privacy protects the confidentiality of thoughts and neural patterns, while cognitive liberty emphasizes freedom from manipulation or coercion over mental processes. Together, these concepts form the foundation of emerging "neurorights" frameworks that seek to safeguard inner mental life in the era of neurotechnology. BCIs blur traditional boundaries between internal experience and observable data. Even noninvasive systems can infer affective states, recognition patterns, or attention levels. Advanced BCIs capable of decoding speech-related or decision-related neural activity could reveal preferences or intentions long before they manifest in behavior. These capabilities introduce the possibility of unwarranted intrusion into the most intimate aspects of human experience.

### 10.4.1 Risks of Cognitive Surveillance and Manipulation

The increasing precision of neuroadaptive algorithms raises concerns about both explicit and subtle forms of cognitive influence. BCIs used in consumer contexts may shape attention patterns or emotional states in ways not fully transparent to users. In clinical or workplace settings, neural monitoring could enable cognitive surveillance, generating pressures to perform or behave in certain ways. Predictive or closed-loop BCIs may not only read neural information but also modulate it, raising questions about autonomy, authenticity of emotional states, and consent to internal influences. Protecting mental privacy therefore requires legal and technical safeguards that prevent monitoring or altering cognitive processes without explicit, voluntary agreement. Ensuring users retain meaningful control over when and how their mental states are shared is essential for preserving autonomy, dignity, and psychological integrity.

## 10.5 Neural Data Governance

Neural data is uniquely sensitive because it can reveal not only what individuals do, but how they think or feel. Unlike conventional biometric data, neural signals enable deep inferences about cognition, emotion, intention, and personality. This requires governance frameworks that classify neural data as a special category of protected information with strict oversight. Effective governance requires well-defined policies for the collection, storage, interpretation, sharing, and deletion of neural data. Users must retain rights to access their neural information, correct inaccuracies, restrict processing, and erase stored data. Because neural signals are meaningful only when processed by ML models, protections must extend to inferred or derived data, not only raw neural recordings.

### 10.5.1 Ownership, Control, and User Rights

A central question concerns who "owns" neural data. Traditional models often assign ownership to device manufacturers or service providers, especially when data is collected on proprietary platforms. However, due to its intimate nature, many scholars argue that neural data should be owned and controlled by the individual. Meaningful user control depends on a robust set of rights governing how neural data is handled throughout its lifecycle. Individuals must be able to access, review, download, and irreversibly delete both their raw neural recordings and any algorithmic inferences derived from them. They should retain the unconditional right to withdraw consent and revoke data processing permissions at any point, without penalty or loss of unrelated services. Equally important is full transparency regarding how their data informs adaptive algorithms or contributes to model training. Finally, strict constraints should apply to any disclosure or transfer of neural data beyond the context for which it was originally collected, particularly with respect to commercial or governmental third parties. Such rights are necessary to prevent users from losing control over information that directly reflects their mental states.

### 10.5.2 Security and Protection Against Misuse

Because neural data can be repurposed for surveillance, profiling, or manipulative applications, strong security protections are essential. Wireless BCIs increase the risk of data interception or malicious interference, making encryption, authentication protocols, and continuous security monitoring critical. As BCIs expand into commercial and consumer markets, regulatory oversight including potentially classifying neural data alongside genetic or health data will be required to prevent misuse for discrimination, behavioral targeting, or psychological profiling.

## 10.6 Commercialization and Corporate Power

Private companies play an increasingly influential role in shaping BCI technologies at the moment, raising concerns about accountability, transparency, and conflicts of interest. Commercial incentives may prioritize rapid deployment, data extraction, or proprietary ecosystems over long-term safety, accessibility, or user autonomy. As the neurotechnology market grows, so does the power imbalance between corporate actors and individual users. One major ethical risk is the commercialization of neural data. Companies may seek to use brain-derived information for product optimization, targeted advertising, or behavioral prediction. Because neural signals can reveal subconscious preferences or emotional responses, commercial exploitation of such data could enable new forms of psychological profiling. Proprietary algorithms obscure how data is processed and analyzed, limiting external scrutiny and accountability. Closed platforms may also restrict interoperability, forcing users to rely on specific corporate ecosystems. This can lead to technological dependency, constrained user choice, and limited transparency about update cycles or firmware changes that affect system behavior.

### 10.6.1 Inequality, Market Concentration, and Neurotechnology Access

Commercialization may deepen existing inequalities if BCI benefits accrue disproportionately to wealthy individuals or well-funded institutions. Advanced BCIs may remain financially inaccessible, creating cognitive or communicative advantages for those who can afford them. Market concentration, where a few corporations control key neurotechnological infrastructures, could exacerbate disparities and reduce public oversight. Responsible commercialization requires transparent data practices, independent audits, and enforceable limits on monetizing neural data. Companies must prioritize user welfare, adopt privacy-preserving design principles, and commit to inclusive access strategies. Collaboration between industry, policymakers, and civil society will be essential to ensure that corporate power aligns with public welfare and that BCI technologies develop in ways that support human autonomy, equality, and dignity.

## 10.7 Neuroethical Guidelines

The question of what can done to minimize the ethical issues raise from BCI technologies. Let's look at the core ethical principles again, which will provide a framework for evaluating the responsible development, deployment, and governance of BCI technologies. While not exhaustive, these principles reflect widely recognized priorities in contemporary neuroethics and are essential for safeguarding user rights, ensuring public trust, and guiding policy formation. Many of these principles are also being actively developed by international organizations (discussed more in later section), which increasingly recognize the need for coordinated global oversight of emerging neurotechnologies (also see Figure 10.1).

- **Security by design:** Given the direct link between brain and device, breaches could cause physical, psychological, or cognitive harm. BCIs must incorporate robust encryption, tamper resistance, continuous monitoring, and fail-safe mechanisms from the outset. Security should not be an optional feature added late in development but a foundational design requirement.
- **User autonomy:** Users must remain in control of how and when BCIs are used. They should be able to withdraw consent, pause or disable the device without penalty, and avoid coercion in clinical, workplace, or consumer contexts. Autonomy also includes control over adaptive or predictive system features, ensuring that BCIs do not override or obscure user intentions.

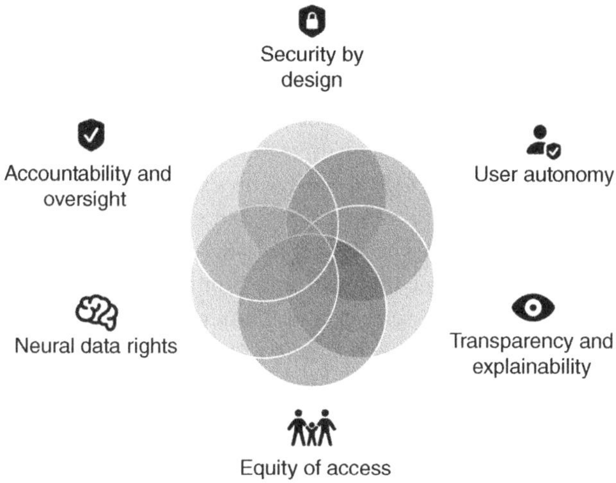


**Figure 10.1** Neuroethics guidelines for responsible development, deployment, and governance.

- **Transparency and explainability:** Systems that rely on AI-based decoding or AI-Copilot must be interpretable to users, clinicians, and regulators. Transparent design includes clear communication of how the system functions, what data it uses, and how algorithmic decisions are generated. This is especially important in contexts such as medical decision-making, legal adjudication, or workplace monitoring, where opaque "black box" models may undermine accountability.
- **Equity of access:** BCI benefits should be distributed fairly across socioeconomic, cultural, and geographic groups. Without deliberate policies and inclusive design strategies, BCIs risk amplifying existing inequalities. Public investment, open research initiatives, and accessible clinical pathways can help ensure that neurotechnology supports social inclusion rather than deepening disparities.
- **Neural data rights:** Neural data is uniquely revealing and must be governed with heightened protection. Users should have meaningful control over their neural information, including the right to access, review, or delete it and the ability to withdraw data-processing permissions at any time. Any sharing or secondary use of neural data should require explicit, informed consent and be subject to strict limitations.
- **Accountability and oversight:** Clear lines of responsibility are essential when BCIs malfunction, produce unintended actions, or generate harmful outcomes. Developers, clinicians, and institutions must be accountable for ensuring safety, reporting adverse events, and maintaining ethical compliance. Independent regulatory bodies should evaluate BCI safety, data practices, and algorithmic fairness, especially as devices become more autonomous or commercialized.

### 10.7.1 International Initiatives

International cooperation will be required to define and harmonize these standards before BCIs become widespread in daily life. Several ongoing multinational initiatives are already working toward this goal. The *OECD* [153] has issued recommendations on responsible neurotechnology innovation, emphasizing safety, transparency, and public trust. *UNESCO* [154] has begun exploring neurotechnology within its broader frameworks for human rights and digital ethics, while the *Council of Europe* [155] is examining whether neurorights such as mental privacy and cognitive liberty, should be incorporated into human rights law. The *Neurorights Foundation* [156] has proposed a global framework for protecting mental integrity and autonomy, and the *World Health Organization* has highlighted the need for governance structures addressing the clinical and public health implications of neurotechnology. The *IEEE Standards Association* has also developed influential ethical guidelines for neurotechnologies as part of its *IEEE Brain* [157] and *Global Initiative on Ethics of Autonomous and Intelligent Systems*, promoting safety, accountability, and human-centered design in emerging neural devices. In parallel, *UNICEF* [158] has initiated work focused on the neuroethical impacts of technology on children, calling for protections tailored to developing brains, child-specific consent models, and safeguards against potentially exploitative uses in educational or consumer contexts. Together, these efforts mark the beginnings of a coordinated international consensus and will be crucial in ensuring that BCIs develop in ways consistent with human dignity, children's rights, and fundamental democratic values.

## 10.8 Practical Implementation

Practical ethics must be embedded in every stage of BCI development, from design to deployment. Institutional Review Board (IRB), clinical ethics committees, and legal advisors should be involved early. Security protocols must be mandatory. Manufacturers should incorporate fail-safes to prevent unintended actions. As BCIs become more autonomous, questions of accountability become more complex. Policymakers and developers must shape new regulations to protect users and promote responsible innovation.

## 10.9 Examples

Let us examine several case studies that illustrate both the promise and peril of BCI technologies as they exist today and how they may shape the future of neural interfaces:

- **Invasive BCI for locked-in patients:** Clinical trials involving invasive BCIs, such as intracortical implants for individuals with locked-in syndrome, have demonstrated remarkable potential to partially restore basic communication. In several instances, patients have been able to convey preferences or emotions through neural signals alone. However, these cases also raise complex ethical questions, particularly around proxy consent. Since some patients may be unable to communicate before implantation, family members or guardians need to make decisions on their behalf. This creates a tension between beneficence of doing what is believed to be in the patient's best interest and respect for autonomy, especially when it is unclear what the patient would choose. These trials underscore the need for ethical protocols that account for impaired consent capacity while safeguarding patient dignity.
- **Neurosecurity threats:** As BCIs become wireless and increasingly integrated into everyday environments, cybersecurity risks escalate. The possibility of unauthorized access to brain data, remote manipulation of neural activity, or malicious signal injection, which is referred to as "brain hacking" [159], poses serious threats to user safety and autonomy. Though currently theoretical, experimental research shows how certain signals could influence motor activity or perception. These risks demand robust technical safeguards, including real-time encryption, authentication protocols, and system redundancy. Just as cybersecurity became central to digital infrastructure, "neurosecurity" is emerging as an essential field for protecting mental integrity and user rights.
- **Lie detection and legal implications:** The use of BCI-based lie detection tools, such as brain fingerprinting and P300 wave detection, has entered courtrooms and law enforcement applications in some jurisdictions [160, 161]. These technologies claim to detect deception or hidden knowledge by analyzing brain responses. However, their scientific validity is contested, and their use raises serious concerns about involuntary self-incrimination, the right to silence, and mental privacy. Courts may soon face decisions about whether brain data can be admitted as legal evidence and whether compelled neural disclosure violates constitutional or human rights. The outcomes of such cases could redefine legal notions of privacy and personhood.
- **Societal stratification and inequality:** As BCI enhancements move beyond therapeutic uses into cognitive or sensory augmentation, access becomes a pressing ethical issue. If only affluent individuals or institutions can afford neural upgrades, a form of cognitive stratification may emerge, leading to a "neuro-divide" between enhanced and non-enhanced populations. This could exacerbate existing educational, economic, and health

inequalities. To address this, governments and international organizations must consider policies for equitable access, such as public funding, open-source platforms, or regulatory caps on enhancement use in competitive settings. Without such measures, BCIs risk reinforcing structural disparities rather than alleviating them.

- **Workplace monitoring and productivity BCIs:** Several companies have begun exploring noninvasive BCIs for monitoring employee attention, stress levels, or fatigue. While marketed as productivity or safety tools, these systems raise significant ethical concerns about cognitive surveillance, coercion, and the erosion of mental privacy in the workplace. Employees may feel pressured to use such tools to remain competitive, even if they are uncomfortable with the degree of monitoring involved. The line between voluntary adoption and implicit coercion becomes blurred, illustrating the need for workplace-specific protections.
- **Educational neurotechnologies for children:** Emerging neurotechnology tools are being piloted in classrooms to monitor concentration or cognitive workload [162]. While intended to support learning, these systems raise profound ethical concerns when applied to children. Developing brains are highly sensitive, and continuous monitoring may create undue pressure, reinforce bias, or affect self-esteem. Questions arise about consent, long-term data storage, and whether such systems normalize intrusive forms of cognitive measurement in educational settings. These examples highlight the need for child-specific neuroethical frameworks.
- **Military applications of BCIs:** Research programs have investigated BCIs for enhancing soldier performance, enabling hands-free operation of devices, or improving situational awareness. While such tools may offer strategic advantages, they raise ethical concerns about coercion, emotional manipulation, and long-term neurological effects. Military hierarchies may pressure soldiers into accepting implants or wearable neurotech, challenging the voluntariness of consent. Additionally, neural data collected in military settings may carry heightened risks of misuse.
- **Consumer neurotechnology and entertainment BCIs:** The rise of consumer grade BCIs used for gaming, meditation, focus training, or smart device control illustrates how rapidly neurotechnology is entering everyday life. However, these devices often operate with minimal regulatory oversight. Companies may collect large volumes of neural data, sometimes without transparent consent or clear data protection practices. The casual nature of

these devices can obscure the sensitivity of the data they gather, raising concerns about commercialization, profiling, and the normalization of neural monitoring.

- **Adaptive BCIs and algorithmic bias:** Many modern BCIs incorporate ML systems that adapt to user behavior over time. While adaptation can improve performance, algorithmic bias can emerge if training data reflects narrow populations. This can lead to unequal access to reliable performance, for example, BCIs that work effectively for certain skin tones, hair types, or neural patterns but not for others. Such biases risk excluding particular demographic groups or reinforcing structural inequities in healthcare and technology.

## 10.10 Summary

As BCIs transition from research to clinical, commercial, educational, and consumer use, the ethical challenges surrounding their deployment have grown increasingly urgent. This chapter outlined the central dimensions of contemporary neuroethics, emphasizing responsible development, informed and inclusive participation, ongoing consent, safety, and equitable access. Public perception and cultural context remain critical, as does understanding how BCIs intersect with identity, agency, and personhood. By acting directly on neural activity, these systems raise questions about autonomy, authenticity, and the protection of mental privacy and cognitive liberty.

Neural data governance has emerged as a defining concern, given the sensitivity of brain-derived information and its potential misuse. Commercialization further complicates these issues, introducing risks related to proprietary algorithms, unequal access, and cognitive surveillance. In response, international organizations including the OECD, UNESCO, WHO, Council of Europe, IEEE, Neurorights Foundation, and UNICEF are developing frameworks to safeguard user rights and promote responsible neurotechnology governance.

Real-world examples from invasive BCIs restoring communication to neurosecurity threats, algorithmic bias, consumer neurotech, and military applications illustrate both the promise of BCIs and the ethical risks they entail. As BCI technologies continue to evolve, robust neuroethical guidance will be essential to ensure that innovation supports human dignity, autonomy, and justice while protecting the most vulnerable.

# 11

# Challenges of Current Neural Interface Technology

Brain–computer interface (BCI) technology is evolving rapidly, driven by advancements in algorithms and artificial intelligence (AI), increasing research into human cognition, and growing interest from private entities and enthusiasts. These factors have contributed to continuous innovation and frequent updates to BCI systems. As discussed in previous chapters, areas such as signal acquisition, neural stimulation, AI and machine learning (ML), and the development of new tools are constantly reshaping the BCI landscape. Despite this progress, broad consumer adoption of BCI technology remains limited. At present, regular use is mostly confined to participants in research studies, individuals with significant medical needs, and a small group of highly dedicated users. Several ongoing challenges, ranging from technical limitations to deeper philosophical and ethical questions, are hindering the transition of BCIs from specialized applications to everyday use. For BCI technology to become a practical part of daily life, whether at home or in the workplace, these challenges must be systematically addressed. Let us examine these challenges and how they may be overcome.

## 11.1 Data Acquisition and Stimulation Challenge

Data acquisition and neural stimulation are fundamental components of BCI systems. However, both present critical challenges that limit their effectiveness in real-world scenarios and hinder broader adoption outside research and clinical settings. Reliable BCIs require stable, high-quality neural signals and precise, controllable stimulation. Yet both invasive and noninvasive approaches face significant limitations in resolution, longevity, comfort, safety, and environmental robustness. These constraints define what is currently feasible and reveal the gap between laboratory grade and everyday BCI applications.

### 11.1.1 Data Acquisition

BCI systems must carefully balance spatial and temporal resolution, signal quality, invasiveness, and ease of use. Invasive methods, such as intracortical microelectrode arrays or electrocorticography (ECoG), offer high-resolution data with excellent bandwidth, making them suitable for fine-grained motor decoding or closed-loop neuromodulation. However, they require neurosurgery, carry medical risks, and suffer from long-term signal degradation due to gliosis, electrode corrosion, and tissue encapsulation. Noninvasive techniques such as electroencephalography (EEG) and functional near-infrared spectroscopy (fNIRS) are safer and more accessible but suffer from lower spatial precision, higher noise, and susceptibility to motion artifacts, limiting their reliability in unconstrained environments. Beyond these fundamental trade-offs, both invasive and noninvasive modalities face further challenges:

- **Motion artifacts and environmental noise:** Everyday environments introduce muscle activity, electrode movement, cable tugging, perspiration, and electromagnetic interference. These factors affect noninvasive systems heavily but also impact implanted systems when external connectors or wireless telemetry are disturbed.
- **Electrode stability and biofouling:** In invasive BCIs, long-term implantation triggers immune responses that gradually degrade electrode performance. Microelectrode arrays may experience reduced spike amplitude, increased impedance, or complete signal loss over months or years.
- **Skin electrode interface limitations:** For noninvasive BCIs, maintaining low impedance contact is difficult across diverse users and activities. Dry electrodes improve usability but often produce higher noise, while wet electrodes require gels that dry over time and require cleaning.
- **Individual neuroanatomical variability:** Skull thickness, cortical folding patterns, vascularization, hair density, and skin properties all influence signal quality. These variations complicate standardized headset design and decoding models.
- **Scalability and practicality:** While high-density invasive systems offer exceptional resolution, power consumption, heat generation, telemetry bandwidth, and surgical complexity severely limit their real-world scalability.

Even the most advanced acquisition systems must navigate these physical, biological, and ergonomic constraints. As a result, current BCIs often face a trade-off where invasive devices achieve high performance but remain clinically restricted, while noninvasive systems are accessible but limited in accuracy and robustness.

### 11.1.2 Stimulation

While stimulation is optional for many BCI applications, it is essential for realizing two-way or closed-loop BCI systems that not only interpret brain activity but also modulate it. These systems are central to neurofeedback, rehabilitation, neuromodulation therapies, and adaptive cognitive enhancement. However, both invasive and noninvasive stimulation face significant limitations. For noninvasive stimulation such as transcranial direct current stimulation (tDCS), transcranial alternating current stimulation (tACS), and transcranial magnetic stimulation (TMS), challenges include:

- **Low spatial specificity:** Current generated by stimulation devices tends to diffuse widely across cortical tissue, activating large regions rather than a well-defined target. This limits the precision of modulation and complicates efforts to influence specific neural circuits.
- **Limited depth penetration:** Most available stimulation is absorbed by the scalp and skull, reducing the amount that reaches the brain. Stimulating deeper structures such as the hippocampus or basal ganglia often requires higher intensities that can cause discomfort or exceed safety thresholds.
- **User discomfort:** Sensations such as tingling, itching, skin heating, phosphenes (flashes of light), and general scalp irritation can occur even at moderate intensities, restricting the range of stimulation parameters that can be safely and comfortably applied.

In invasive stimulation approaches such as deep brain stimulation (DBS), cortical microstimulation, challenges include:

- **Surgical risks and long-term maintenance:** Infection, hardware failure, lead migration, and the need for battery replacements or device revisions.
- **Neural plasticity effects:** Chronic stimulation can alter local circuits in unpredictable ways, affecting cognition, or mood.
- **Surgical risks and long-term maintenance:** Most of these implantation procedures carry risks of infection, hemorrhage, hardware failure, and lead migration. Over time, implanted devices may require battery replacements, software updates, or surgical revisions, adding to the overall clinical burden.
- **Neural plasticity effects:** A continuous stimulation for long-term could augment neural circuits, sometimes producing therapeutic benefits but also creating unintended alterations in cognition, emotion, or behavior. These adaptive responses remain difficult to predict or fully control.
- **Parameter optimization:** There is lack of understanding on identifying the optimal stimulation amplitude, frequency, pulse shape, and timing. Individual variability in anatomy and neural responsiveness makes personalized tuning complex and often reliant on labor-intensive trial-and-error methods.

Both invasive and noninvasive approaches struggle with dynamic responsiveness. Closed-loop systems must adapt stimulation based on real-time neural feedback, yet neural states shift rapidly, demanding fast, precise control algorithms that remain safe across a variety of contexts.

### 11.1.3 Integration of Acquisition and Stimulation

Combining acquisition and stimulation into a single closed-loop system introduces additional layers of complexity. Stimulation pulses often generate large artifacts that obscure or overwhelm concurrent neural recordings, particularly when acquisition and stimulation are delivered in nearby cortical regions. Addressing this challenge requires sophisticated artifact suppression methods, careful hardware isolation, and precisely timed control strategies that can separate true neural activity from stimulation-induced noise. In implantable systems, integration also heightens concerns related to heat generation, power consumption, device miniaturization, wireless telemetry bandwidth, and long-term biocompatibility. For wearable systems, combining acquisition and stimulation complicates mechanical design, as headsets must maintain stable electrode contact, minimize movement-related disturbances, and remain comfortable enough for prolonged daily use. Achieving reliable integration therefore requires advances in both hardware and algorithmic design. To make BCI systems viable for everyday use, future developments will need to deliver high-fidelity neural acquisition coupled with precise, user-friendly stimulation methods that are safe, durable, and adaptable across diverse real-world environments. Overcoming these scientific and engineering barriers is essential for transitioning BCI technologies from controlled laboratory settings into seamless, daily-life applications.

## 11.2 Technological Challenge

Despite significant advancements, robust and reliable BCI systems are still largely limited to specific paradigms, such as motor imagery (MI), which tend to be more resilient to interference from concurrent cognitive processes. However, brain signals are inherently variable, even under controlled conditions. BCI systems face intra-, inter-, and nonstationarity in signals due to mental and emotional states as well as surrounding environmental factors such as electrical noise. For example, over the course of a single BCI session, a user may begin with high motivation and focus but gradually experience fatigue, boredom, or cognitive overload. These shifts can dramatically alter neural signals, reducing the accuracy and responsiveness of BCI systems. Although Chapter 7 explores potential approaches to mitigate these issues, such as incorporating adaptive interfaces and game mechanics, these strategies remain in early stages of development and present substantial implementation challenges.

### 11.2.1 Cognitive and Contextual Variability

A major source of technological complexity in BCI lies in our limited understanding of how ongoing cognitive processes influence signal patterns. As discussed in Chapter 7, mental states such as fatigue, stress, mental workload, anxiety, mind wandering, distraction, and frustration can dynamically modulate the neural signals that BCI systems rely upon. This variability makes it difficult to maintain consistent performance across different users and usage contexts. Without a comprehensive understanding of these influences, BCI systems remain highly vulnerable to context-induced degradation. For instance, an algorithm trained on a user in a calm, focused state may perform poorly when that same user is under stress or cognitive load.

### 11.2.2 Need for Adaptive and Personalized Systems

To address these challenges, future BCI systems must integrate:

- **Longitudinal user modeling:** Continuously tracking cognitive and neural patterns over extended periods to develop more robust and personalized user profiles. In this context, take-home BCI kits can be particularly useful for enabling long-term data collection in naturalistic environments.
- **Context-aware signal processing:** Detecting and compensating for contextual variability and noise in real time. Incorporating multimodal data sources such as physiological signals or environmental sensors can help BCI systems better interpret contextual information and enhance signal quality, thereby improving the signal-to-noise ratio (SNR).
- **Adaptive machine learning:** Implementing models that dynamically adjust to changes in a user's cognitive and emotional states. These algorithms continuously refine their predictions as they accumulate user-specific data, leading to more reliable and responsive BCI performance.

### 11.2.3 Challenges in Real-world Deployment

Implementing these adaptive systems introduces its own set of technical hurdles:

- **Data scarcity and annotation:** Real-time identification of cognitive states depends on large volumes of annotated data, which is expensive, time-consuming, and difficult to obtain at scale. To address this, researchers are exploring the development of large-scale neural activity models that aim to generalize across tasks and individuals, potentially enabling unified or pre-trained models with minimal fine-tuning.

- **Computational overhead:** Adaptive algorithms must process data and adjust system behavior in real time while maintaining low latency and minimizing hardware demands. Balancing algorithmic complexity with responsiveness is a persistent technical challenge, especially in mobile or embedded BCI systems.
- **Generalization across users:** Creating models that adapt effectively without overfitting to individual users is an ongoing research problem. Inter-subject variability in brain signals remains high, and current models often require extensive user-specific calibration, limiting scalability and usability.
- **Integration with user interfaces:** Effective integration of adaptive algorithms with user interfaces requires intuitive, real-time feedback mechanisms that support user engagement without being distracting or intrusive. Designing such interfaces is critical to maintaining usability and system transparency.

## 11.3 Ethical Challenge

Technical challenges aside, ethical concerns pose significant barriers to the widespread adoption of BCIs. A major issue involves data privacy and the responsible use of neural information. Brain data collected via BCIs could be used not only to optimize device performance but also for secondary purposes such as targeted advertising, behavioral prediction, or even cognitive profiling, often without explicit or informed user consent.

These issues raise profound concerns about mental privacy, autonomy, and the potential misuse of cognitive data. There have been active efforts in this direction by various state authorities, as discussed in Chapter 10. Some of the key challenges are as follows:

### 11.3.1 Privacy and Data Ownership

One of the central ethical questions and challenges for BCI systems entering the general public for regular everyday use concerns brain data ownership. Current approaches do not adequately address brain data ownership. Most off-the-shelf consumer products either store data within the device or on cloud servers owned by service providers, enabling them to store, analyze, and potentially monetize user data. However, brain data is highly sensitive in nature; therefore, stronger protections are required. An unauthorized access to neural data could lead to unprecedented forms of exploitation, manipulation, or discrimination now as well as in the future. Such data can be combined with existing behavioral data by data brokers to further enhance algorithmic predictability and exploit users. For example, subtle patterns in EEG signals could theoretically be used to infer political preferences, susceptibility to certain diseases, or aspects of personality, raising serious implications for individual freedoms and rights.

### 11.3.2 Workplace and Institutional Use

Ethical concerns become even more acute when BCIs are deployed in institutional settings, such as workplaces, schools, or healthcare environments. In a workplace, employees may feel coerced into using BCIs to monitor productivity, cognitive load, or stress levels. Although intended to optimize work processes, such monitoring risks undermining autonomy, creating new forms of surveillance, and exacerbating power imbalances between employers and employees. The potential misuse of BCI technologies could lead to subtle but significant shifts in workplace dynamics, where employees are judged or penalized based on real or perceived cognitive states. Similar concerns extend to educational settings, where BCI technologies could be used to monitor student attention or emotional engagement, raising questions about consent, fairness, and the potential psychological impact on young users.

### 11.3.3 Vulnerable Populations and Consent

Particular care must be taken when considering the use of BCI technologies in vulnerable populations, such as children, individuals with cognitive impairments, or patients undergoing treatment. Informed consent in these groups is particularly complex, as individuals may not fully understand the scope and risks associated with BCI data collection and use. Additionally, parental or institutional consent for children raises difficult questions about long-term impacts on privacy and autonomy. Decisions made on behalf of minors today could have unforeseen consequences decades later if neural data is stored, shared, or repurposed. Addressing these ethical challenges requires more than technical solutions; it demands proactive policy development, public dialogue, and interdisciplinary collaboration.

## 11.4 Design Challenge

Perhaps one of the most underestimated yet crucial challenges for the future of BCI technology lies in device design and form factor. While there is significant interest in using BCIs for various applications, many current devices fail to meet user expectations regarding comfort, usability, and aesthetics. Most existing BCI headsets prioritize technical performance but often overlook how a device feels and looks when worn in everyday settings. From a user's perspective, wearable technology should seamlessly integrate into daily life, similar to popular consumer products like headphones, smartwatches, or smart glasses. However, BCI headsets are often bulky, visually intrusive, or uncomfortable, resembling research prototypes rather than consumer-ready products. For example, while full-head headphones are accepted in public, helmet-like, or rigid BCI designs are socially awkward and discourage broader use.

Design is not just about aesthetics or user acceptance; it also directly impacts the technical performance of BCIs. A well-designed, ergonomically fitted device can significantly improve the quality of neural signal acquisition by maintaining stable electrode contact, reducing movement artifacts, and enhancing overall SNR. In contrast, poorly designed systems are prone to electrode displacement, leading to signal degradation and user frustration. Future BCI devices must therefore meet multiple criteria simultaneously: they must be lightweight, discreet, easy to wear, durable, and capable of maintaining high-quality neural signal acquisition and stimulation across a variety of environments. Achieving this requires interdisciplinary collaboration between neuroscientists, engineers, designers, and material scientists. Advances in flexible electronics, biocompatible materials, and miniaturized sensors offer promising avenues toward creating the next generation of BCIs that are both effective and user-friendly.

Moreover, personalization may become a key aspect of future BCI design. Individual differences in head shape, hair type, skin properties, and daily activities necessitate adjustable, customizable devices to ensure comfort and consistent performance across diverse users. In this context, modular designs, self-adjusting electrode systems, and even smart fabrics could play significant roles. While this challenge may be a lower priority compared to other fundamental requirements, it remains critical for transitioning BCI technology from specialized laboratories and clinical settings into the hands of everyday users at home, work, and beyond.

## 11.5 Standardization and Interoperability Challenge

As BCI technology continues to evolve but remains highly interdisciplinary in nature, another significant challenge lies in the lack of standardized protocols and interoperability across devices, software platforms, and data formats. Current BCI research, conducted by individuals from a variety of fields, is highly fragmented. Different researchers, laboratories, organizations, companies, and open-source communities often use proprietary formats for data collection, device communication, and algorithmic implementation. This fragmentation hinders collaboration, slows innovation, and creates barriers for users and developers alike.

### 11.5.1 Lack of Unified Data Standards

There is no universally accepted format for neural data, making it difficult to share datasets, compare models, or reproduce experimental results [157]. This limits the effectiveness of cross-study analyses and large-scale benchmarking of BCI algorithms. As the field matures, the establishment of open standards for BCI data similar to those in genomics or medical imaging (e.g., DICOM) is essential for accelerating progress.

### 11.5.2 Device and Platform Compatibility

Interoperability across BCI devices and platforms is still in its infancy. Most systems are tightly coupled to specific hardware or software stacks, preventing users from mixing and matching components to suit their needs. For example, a researcher may not be able to use a preferred signal processing tool with a commercial headset due to closed application programming interfaces (APIs) or licensing restrictions. This lack of compatibility limits user choice and innovation.

### 11.5.3 Call for Regulatory and Industrial Collaboration

Solving this issue requires active collaboration between industry stakeholders, academic institutions, and regulatory bodies to define open protocols, encourage data sharing, and establish best practices. Standardization would not only foster innovation but also build trust in the safety, quality, and reliability of BCI technologies.

## 11.6 Reliability, Robustness, and Real-world Deployment Challenge

A major barrier to everyday BCI adoption lies in the difficulty of maintaining reliable performance in real-world environments. While many BCIs perform well in laboratory settings, their accuracy declines sharply when used outside controlled conditions. Factors such as body movement, sweating, changes in temperature, electrode displacement, and environmental electromagnetic interference can cause substantial signal degradation. Even small variations in electrode contact or user posture can reduce SNR and disrupt decoding performance. These challenges reflect the intrinsic fragility of neural signals. In practice, BCI systems should be able to operate in diverse and unpredictable environments during physical activity, over long periods, in outdoor settings, or while users multitask. Ensuring robustness under such conditions requires new methods in sensor engineering, adaptive noise reduction, and fault-tolerant algorithms. Without these advances, BCI systems will remain limited to short, supervised sessions rather than seamless integration into daily life.

## 11.7 Usability and Human Factors Challenge

Even when technological performance is adequate, many BCIs fail to meet user expectations for everyday usability. Current devices frequently impose significant setup time, require electrode preparation, or depend on skilled operators unless invasive. Noninvasive headsets may need careful positioning, recalibration, or maintenance that discourages regular use. In addition, long-term wearability remains a major challenge because headbands or electrode caps can be heavy, uncomfortable, or prone to slipping during movement.

Additionally, human factors play a central role in whether BCIs become practical consumer technologies. Users expect devices that are intuitive, quick to set up, comfortable for long periods, and easy to maintain. For noninvasive BCIs, hygiene concerns such as cleaning electrodes, managing gels, or sharing headsets remain significant barriers in both home and institutional settings. Although wearable formats similar to headphones or earbuds are socially acceptable, current BCI hardware often lacks equivalent comfort, stability, and convenience. For implantable BCIs, human factors take a different form, including surgical burdens, long-term care of implanted components, and the need to minimize discomfort or lifestyle restrictions. Addressing these issues will require a significant shift toward ergonomic, user-centered design and minimal-maintenance systems that support continuous, everyday use across both wearable and implantable form factors.

## 11.8 Calibration and Training Challenge

BCI systems often require extensive calibration before they can be used effectively. MI BCIs, for example, may demand lengthy sessions to collect training data during which users must repeatedly imagine specific motor movements. Calibration must frequently be repeated before each session due to signal drift, nonstationarity, or changes in physiological state. This requirement for frequent recalibration reduces practicality and discourages adoption. User training is also a significant challenge. Novice users may struggle to generate consistent neural patterns, and some individuals referred to as "BCI-illiterate" cannot achieve sufficient control despite training. Reducing or eliminating calibration, enabling rapid onboarding, and developing models that generalize across users remain active areas of research. Plug-and-play BCIs will require advances in transfer learning, subject-independent models, and real-time adaptive decoding.

## 11.9 Long-term Safety and Physiological Impact Challenge

Long-term use of BCIs raises concerns about safety and physiological effects, particularly for implantable and wearable systems. In invasive devices, scar tissue (gliosis) can gradually form around electrodes, degrading signal quality and requiring replacement surgery. Implants also carry risks of infection, mechanical failure, or tissue damage. For wearable systems, prolonged electrode contact can lead to skin irritation, pressure points, or discomfort.

Additionally, closed-loop stimulation systems may alter neural plasticity over time in ways that are not yet fully understood. Repeated stimulation of certain brain regions could produce unintended long-term consequences for cognition, emotion, or motor function. Ensuring long-term biocompatibility, minimizing adverse effects, and establishing safety standards for chronic BCI use remain essential steps before BCIs can be trusted for widespread daily deployment.

## 11.10 Psychological and Cognitive Load Challenge

BCI use can impose substantial cognitive and emotional demands on users. Many systems require sustained attention, precise MI, or continuous monitoring of feedback. Over time, this can lead to cognitive fatigue, frustration, or performance decline. Users may also experience stress or anxiety when systems misinterpret intentions or fail unpredictably, undermining the sense of agency and control.

Certain BCIs, particularly those involving stimulation, may influence mood, arousal, or emotional responses, creating further psychological complexity. Understanding the cognitive burden of interacting with BCIs and designing interfaces that minimize psychological strain is essential to ensuring user well-being and long-term engagement. This challenge highlights the need for interdisciplinary research integrating cognitive science, human–computer interaction (HCI), and affective neuroscience.

## 11.11 Social Acceptance and Trust Challenge

Even when BCIs are technically functional and safe, social acceptance remains a major obstacle. Many individuals express discomfort with technologies that interface with the brain, fearing "mind reading," loss of control, or data misuse, as outlined in Chapter 10. Public understanding of BCIs is limited, and misconceptions are widespread. Additionally, devices that look unusual or invasive may create social stigma or discourage use in public spaces.

Trust in companies and institutions also plays a critical role. Concerns about corporate surveillance, neural data collection, and opaque algorithms may deter potential users. Ethical controversies such as the use of BCIs in the workplace for monitoring attention or stress can further undermine public confidence. Building trust will require transparent communication about capabilities and limitations, user-centered design, and strong governance frameworks that protect autonomy and privacy.

**Table 11.1** Challenges in BCI applications and its key issues.

| Challenge category | Key issues |
|---|---|
| Data Acquisition & Stimulation | Low SNR, bulky hardware, and imprecise stimulation |
| Technological | Cognitive variability, real-time adaptation, and algorithm robustness |
| Ethical | Privacy, consent, and workplace surveillance |
| Design | Usability, comfort, aesthetics, and personalization |
| Standardization | Data formats, device compatibility, and lack of protocols |

## 11.12 Summary

The development of BCI technology represents a frontier in cognitive neuroscience and HCI with vast potential across healthcare, education, entertainment, and beyond. However, this potential remains largely untapped due to a wide range of technological, ethical, cognitive, and practical challenges. Key obstacles include the difficulty of acquiring clean, reliable neural signals in real-world environments, the limited precision and safety of current stimulation techniques, and the complex interplay between brain activity and constantly shifting cognitive states. Further complicating this landscape are issues of user interface design, ethical risks involving neural data privacy, and the lack of standardization that restricts interoperability and scalability. Also see Table 11.1 which summarize these issues.

Overcoming these barriers demands a multidisciplinary effort. Advances in neuroscience, AI, engineering, materials science, ethics, and user-centered design must converge to make BCI systems practical, safe, and accessible. While the road ahead is long, incremental progress in adaptive algorithms, user-friendly hardware, and ethical frameworks will be essential to bringing BCI technology from the lab into daily life. By addressing these challenges holistically, the future of BCIs can move from niche use cases to a transformative tool that empowers individuals and augments human capability in everyday settings.

# 12

# Envisioning the Future of Brain–Computer Interfaces

The idea of controlling machines from thoughts sounds like science fiction or belong to the world of superheroes; yet current progress and development in BCI have shown this is not a distant future but a emerging possibility now. In fact, every idea we entertain, every memory we recall, and every action we take, and every word I wrote here, is essentially originated in the brain through electrical and chemical processes. This makes the brain the most private and intimate space but also a highly sophisticated computational system. Therefore, it is no surprise that researchers, scientists, philosophers, and writers are so fascinated with this organ. Current progress is merely a scratch on the surface of understanding this organ, and the BCIs of simple control to speech reconstruction is already showing remarkable progress that signals what lies ahead. However, realizing the bold advances in the BCI requires significant progress in neuroscience, materials science, signal processing, machine learning (ML), and neuroethical guardrails. These current hurdles may become stepping stones in the near future for rapid innovation in BCI. This chapter examines where this path may lead to and outlines the future across four time horizons, as shown in Table 12.1, in which BCIs could reshape communication, medicine, creativity, and even our sense of self.

**Table 12.1** Future of BCI and its focus.

| Section | Time horizon | Focus area |
|---|---|---|
| The Near Future | 5–10 years | Usability, clinical utility, and consumer BCI |
| Foundational Milestones | 10–15 years | Core technology breakthroughs |
| Strategic Innovations | 10–30 years | Infrastructure, scalability, and ethics |
| Beyond the Horizon | 30–50+ years | Societal transformation, speculative futures |

## 12.1 The Near Future: Practical Expectations for BCIs

BCIs have already demonstrated their potential to revolutionize the way we interact with technology. From enabling control of external devices to decoding inner thoughts such as speech and visual imagery, the scope of applications continues to expand. They are being explored not only for clinical use, medical diagnosis, and therapy but also for enhancing user experiences in entertainment, gaming, and personalized technology. However, most current BCI applications are still in their early stages and are not yet mature enough for widespread consumer adoption, some of the challenges behind this are discussed in Chapter 10. The immediate future of BCI, therefore, involves refining and stabilizing these innovations to allow smooth integration into daily life. A major goal should be to develop systems that can assist individuals with routine tasks, restore lost abilities, and potentially enhance cognitive functions. For instance, speech reconstruction through BCIs holds the promise of digitally restoring communication for individuals with speech impairments, offering them a new level of independence. Similarly, control strategies based on mental imagery are showing reliable results, particularly in clinical and research settings involving direct brain recordings. The next important step is to adapt these technologies for safe and effective use outside controlled environments. This section discussed on developments expected within the next 5–10 years and highlighting current prototypes maturing into practical, usable tools. Some key expectations for BCI include:

### 12.1.1 Development of Novel Sensing Technologies, Both Invasive and Noninvasive

There is active research in the field of sensing technologies to capture brain signals. These research efforts aim to design new sensing methods that could offer greater precision, reliability, and long-term stability in capturing brain signals. Among them, invasive sensing techniques aim to provide high-resolution data from deeper parts of the brain using implanted electrodes. On the other hand, noninvasive approaches, including wearable EEG devices and emerging techniques based on optical imaging or focused ultrasound, are being developed to offer safer and portable alternatives without requiring surgery. These innovations will not only enhance the accuracy of brain signal acquisition but will also expand access to BCI technologies. In parallel, there is also growing interest in stimulation-based BCI systems, where electrical, magnetic, or optical signals are sent back to the brain, enabling two-way interaction in BCI. Such bidirectional BCI systems could support applications like sensory feedback in prosthetics or modulation of cognitive states, making BCIs more interactive and responsive.

### 12.1.2 Improved Information Transfer Rates Between Brain and Device

One of the key limitations in current BCI systems is the relatively low rate of communication between the brain and external devices. Unlike speech and typing, which allow fast and expressive communication, BCIs still struggle with a relatively low information transfer rate due to slow signal interpretation. There is active research in this area aimed at developing fast, reliable, and responsive BCIs. A fast or with a high information transfer rate BCI, would offer more fluid and natural interaction with the environment and enable the real-time communication, complex control of robotic limbs, and interaction with immersive environments. Therefore, BCIs in the future will enable high speed interaction in both clinical and everyday settings.

### 12.1.3 Integration of Advanced ML Algorithms for Better Decoding Accuracy

Accurately translating brain activity into commands requires advanced neural decoding techniques. ML, particularly deep learning and adaptive models, is playing a critical role in this process. These algorithms have shown to learn from the unique brain activity patterns of each user, adapt over time, and even compensate for variations in signal quality or mental state. By continuously improving decoding accuracy, ML may reduce the need for manual calibration and extensive training, making BCIs more practical and efficient. Furthermore, combining decoding with real-time feedback and stimulation opens the door to closed-loop systems, where the brain and device continuously inform and influence each other.

### 12.1.4 Introduction of User-friendly BCI Solutions in the Consumer Market

There has been significant progress in BCI, which will continue to evolve; however, there is still a disconnect between BCI technology and consumers. To minimize this gap, there is a need to design BCI systems that are not only very accurate but also very easy to use, affordable, and portable. Researchers and developers in the industry are also working on simplify interfaces, minimize setup time, and improve device portability. These steps will ensure that users without technical knowledge and expertise can directly benefit from BCI. Consumer applications may include health monitoring, immersive gaming, personalized control of digital environments, and cognitive enhancement tools. A major factor in this transition is public acceptance, which depends on trust, ethical design, and perceived value. Creating BCI systems that are both functional and approachable will be essential for their successful adoption in everyday life.

## 12.2 Foundational Milestones in BCI Technology

This section outlines the key technical breakthroughs and research frontiers that may be achieved in the medium term (10–15 years) and will enable more advanced BCI capabilities. As the field continues to mature, the next generation of progress will depend on a convergence of technological innovation, clinical validation, ethical governance, and user-centered design. These milestones are interconnected and represent the steps required to transition BCIs from experimental systems to reliable, safe, and widely adopted technologies across healthcare, education, communication, and human augmentation. In the following pages, we examine the developments that are most critical for this transition.

### 12.2.1 Reliable Noninvasive Brain Signal Acquisition

One of the primary goals in BCI development is to capture high-quality brain signals without requiring invasive surgery. Achieving this involves advances in sensor design, materials science, and signal amplification techniques. Emerging technologies such as optically pumped magnetometer magnetoencephalography (OPM-MEG) [55], ultra-high-density electroencephalography (EEG) arrays, and functional near-infrared spectroscopy (fNIRS) are being explored for this purpose. Additionally, improvements in noise reduction, dry electrodes, and motion artifact compensation will be critical for enabling long-term, comfortable, and unobtrusive brain monitoring in real-world environments.

### 12.2.2 Real-time Neural Decoding of Complex Cognitive and Emotional States

Future BCIs must move beyond decoding basic cognitive functions such as motor intentions and focus on understanding more abstract cognitive states such as attention, memory recall, decision-making, and emotion. To reach such a goal, massive annotated neural datasets, multimodal neural embeddings, and self-supervised learning approaches that can decode mental states across users and contexts are required. Decoding mental states could fuel applications related to adaptive user interfaces, mental health diagnostics, emotion-aware virtual assistance, dynamic learning environments, etc.

### 12.2.3 Closed-loop and Adaptive BCI Systems with Integrated Stimulation

Closed-loop, or two-way, BCI systems represent a major evolution in the field by enabling bidirectional interaction between the brain and external devices. These systems not only record neural activity but also deliver targeted stimulation in response, creating a dynamic feedback loop. Stimulation modalities including transcranial magnetic stimulation (TMS), transcranial direct current stimulation (tDCS), focused ultrasound, and optogenetic technologies remain largely non-portable and are currently accessible primarily in research or clinical settings. These systems hold promise for more precise modulation of brain function.

Building on this foundation, closed-loop architectures already support interventions such as the suppression of pathological activity in epilepsy and the facilitation of motor recovery in clinical rehabilitation. They are also being explored for cognitive enhancement, where real-time coupling between neural signals and stimulation may improve learning and memory in controlled settings.

### 12.2.4 Next-generation Implantable BCIs and Neuromodulation Devices

While invasive BCIs provide high signal fidelity, they must overcome challenges related to tissue compatibility, long-term stability, and surgical complexity. Future systems aim to be less intrusive, incorporating flexible bioelectronics, biocompatible coatings, wireless communication, and self-powered operation. Nanotechnology-enabled implants and injectable neural dust [163] are promising directions. Moreover, implantable devices are increasingly being designed not only for signal acquisition but also for direct stimulation of brain tissue. These include DBS systems for Parkinson's disease, cortical implants for visual restoration, and hippocampal prosthetics for memory support. The convergence of sensing and stimulation in a single platform is essential for building intelligent neuroprosthetic systems.

### 12.2.5 Multimodal and Context-aware BCI Systems

Integrating brain activity with other physiological, behavioral, and environmental data streams can significantly improve accuracy and contextual awareness. Future systems will combine EEG, MEG or invasive signals with eye-tracking, speech analysis, electromyography (EMG), galvanic skin response, and ambient sensors. In stimulation contexts, this multimodal input can dynamically adjust the timing and intensity of neural feedback to optimize learning, attention, or rehabilitation. Such systems can be used in neuroadaptive gaming, assistive technology, or real-time stress management.

### 12.2.6 Neural Digital Twins and Personalized Neurostimulation Models

A highly promising direction involves the creation of neural digital twins such that computational and foundational models that simulate an individual's brain structure and function in real time. These models can be used to predict how the brain will respond to stimulation, tailor BCI decoding algorithms, or simulate outcomes of medical interventions. Combined with personalized neurostimulation protocols, digital twins could enable targeted treatments for mood disorders, cognitive decline, or chronic pain. This convergence of neuroscience, bioinformatics, and AI represents a key milestone toward precision neurotechnology.

### 12.2.7 User-centered Design, Accessibility, and Inclusivity

Future BCI systems are expected to place much stronger emphasis on usability, comfort, and inclusivity so that they can support everyday use across diverse settings. Progress in ergonomic hardware, intuitive interfaces, rapid calibration, and low maintenance operation will be central to making BCIs more practical and widely adoptable. Cloud-based platforms may support these developments by enabling remote setup, diagnostics, and personalized adjustments tailored to individual users. A user-centered design will play a crucial role in ensuring that BCIs effectively serve the populations who can benefit most, including individuals with motor impairments, neurodegenerative conditions, or learning disabilities. Inclusivity will also require careful consideration of cultural, economic, and geographic diversity so that advances in BCI technology contribute to broader access rather than widening existing disparities.

### 12.2.8 Standardization, Privacy, and Ethical Governance

As BCI systems grow in complexity and scope, there is a pressing need for global standards that define data formats, safety protocols, clinical trial procedures, and ethical boundaries. These standards will ensure device interoperability, enable transparent benchmarking, and protect user data from misuse while helping scientist and researchers to collaborate [157]. Ethical governance must address emerging issues such as mental privacy, consent in continuous monitoring, neurosecurity against external manipulation, and equitable access. Stimulation-based BCIs especially require rigorous ethical scrutiny, as modulating brain activity directly can alter perception, mood, and behavior.

These milestones together form the roadmap toward an intelligent, adaptive, and socially integrated BCI future. The transition from lab-based systems to practical tools that can augment human capabilities, restore lost functions, and foster new forms of communication is well underway. Continued collaboration across neuroscience, engineering, medicine, and ethics will be vital in shaping a future where BCI and stimulation technologies become safe, transformative, and accessible to all. Chapter 10 discussed these issues more in detail.

## 12.3 Innovations Needed and Looking Ahead

To fully realize the transformative potential of BCIs over the coming decades, a broad set of innovations will be required spanning advanced materials, computational architectures, sensing technologies, biological engineering, and the design of human-centered systems. These developments go beyond incremental improvements; these innovations will represent the cross-disciplinary foundation on which next-generation BCIs will be built. The convergence of these fields will shape systems that are more precise, adaptive, scalable, and deeply integrated into everyday life. Let's look some of key ones needed:

### 12.3.1 Breakthroughs in Materials Science for Neural Interfaces

Future BCIs will rely on ultra-thin, flexible, and biocompatible materials that conform seamlessly to neural tissue while minimizing inflammation or scarring. Advances in conductive polymers and organic electrochemical transistors [164], long-term stable electronic dura mater interfaces [165], and stretchable bioelectronics [166] will enable high-fidelity, durable sensing, and stimulation. Emerging materials such as graphene meshes, MXenes, and OECT-based biotransistors promise enhanced conductivity, biostability, and mechanical resilience. Collectively, these innovations will support dense sensor arrays for high-resolution neural recording and enable minimally invasive implantation through injectable, flexible, or unfolding structures.

### 12.3.2 Miniaturized, Wearable, and Implantable Systems

Beyond clinical settings, a widespread adoption of BCI requires an improvement in portability and comfort. There has been progress in miniaturized amplifiers and foldable high-density electrodes [167], conformal energy-harvesting technologies [168], and injectable nanoscale systems such as neural dust [163]. They will support an unobtrusive and continuous neural interface, suitable for widespread adoptation. Battery-free or energy harvesting designs including piezoelectric, inductive, and biochemical power systems will further reduce maintenance demands, enabling long-term, seamless operation without tethering users to external hardware.

### 12.3.3 Quantum and Ultra-sensitive Neural Sensing

Quantum magnetometers [169], optical magnetometry-based devices [170], and other quantum enhanced sensing technologies [58] offer unmatched sensitivity to the weak magnetic fields generated by neural activity. These devices may soon enable noninvasive measurements with spatial resolutions approaching those of invasive implants and replace dominate over EEG. Such advances could lead to lightweight helmets, wearable quantum MEG (qMEG) headsets, and other compact systems capable of recording deep brain dynamics relevant to cognition, emotion, and memory.

### 12.3.4 Advanced AI and Neuromorphic Computing for Real-time Decoding

Future BCIs will depend on multimodal AI architectures capable of integrating neural, behavioral, and contextual signals. Latent dynamical systems and related methods [171] promise more robust decoding, while neuromorphic processors such as Intel's Loihi [172] provide low-power, real-time on-device computation. Breakthroughs in high-performance decoding such as imagined handwriting interfaces [173] illustrate the potential for highly adaptive, personalized BCIs that evolve continuously with the user's neural patterns.

### 12.3.5 Synthetic Biology and Neural Circuit Engineering

Synthetic biology is enabling next-generation interfaces that integrate biological and digital functionality at the cellular and molecular levels. Optogenetic actuators and cell specific targeting strategies, nanoscale mapping technologies like expansion microscopy [174], and engineered ion channels or neuromodulation circuits support precise read/write access to neural pathways. These tools open new possibilities for self-repairing interfaces, long-term stability, and programmable modulation of perception, cognition, and memory.

### 12.3.6 Optical and Holographic Neural Modulation

Optical stimulation approaches including scanless holographic optogenetics [175], holographic photostimulation, and two-photon holographic excitation could provide high-resolution, contactless modulation of targeted neural populations. Advances in fiber optic microstructures, waveguides, and minimally invasive light-emitting devices may enable cortical modulation even through the skull. These developments hold promise for applications in sensory restoration, cognitive enhancement, and adaptive neuromodulation.

### 12.3.7 Scalable Infrastructure for Neural Data

As BCIs evolve, they will generate continuous, high-bandwidth neural data streams requiring scalable, efficient computational infrastructures. High-density platforms such as Neuropixels [176], combined with insights from large-scale neuroscience initiatives, will drive the development of neuromorphic accelerators and hybrid cloud–edge architectures. Standardized pipelines for real-time processing, synchronization, and secure encoding will be essential for long-term, distributed BCI ecosystems.

### 12.3.8 Interdisciplinary Collaboration and Co-design

The future of BCIs will be shaped by collaboration across neuroscience, AI, biomedical engineering, cognitive science, ethics, and design. Interdisciplinary frameworks and integration with human–computer interaction methodologies will help ensure that BCIs are matched to biological constraints and real-world contexts. Co-design approaches involving engineers, clinicians, and end-users from early development stages are critical for ensuring usability, feasibility, and acceptance.

### 12.3.9 Human-centered Design and User Experience Optimization

To bring BCIs for long-term use and adoption in everyday life, there is a need for a strong emphasis on human cognitive, emotional, and ergonomic needs. Additionally, such BCIs also need highly accurate classification, adaptive algorithms, and user-centered design principles to allow intuitive interaction with low cognitive load and personalized presentation. These principles and improvements will promote trust and sustained engagement with BCIs in daily life.

As these principles, technologies, and system-level innovations mature, BCIs applications will extend beyond therapeutic and assistive need to more toward augmenting core aspects of human cognition. Future interfaces may support enhanced memory, expanded attentional capacity, emotional regulation, deeper immersion in digital environments, and even direct brain-to-brain communication. These advancements will serve as the foundation for the long-term evolution of BCIs toward integrated, adaptive, and cognitively transformative systems.

## 12.4 Beyond the Horizon: The Next 50 Years of BCI

Looking 50 years ahead, the boundary between human and machine cognition may be blurred significantly, and we may see a potential future world where human and machine converge into a unified cognitive continuum. BCIs are expected to evolve beyond their current role as assistive technologies and become embedded neural coprocessors augmenting, complementing, and potentially transforming the way we think, learn, and communicate. As this integration deepens, BCIs may fundamentally alter human capabilities and challenge long-standing distinctions between biology and AI. Future BCI systems may be capable of extending memory capacity with artificial ones, accelerating learning, enhancing decision-making processes, and decoding abstract thoughts and emotional states with high precision. Such developments would not merely support human cognition but actively co-shape it, enabling real-time optimization of mental performance across diverse contexts.

One particularly transformative concept is that of direct brain-to-brain communication. This can be referred to as a *brainnet*; this capability would allow individuals to share raw sensory experiences, emotions, and cognitive states without the mediation of language. The emergence of such a network could redefine human collaboration, fostering unprecedented levels of empathy, mutual understanding, and collective problem-solving.

Another potential future speculation with BCI could be the digital replication or transfer of consciousness, commonly termed *mind uploading* by futurists in popular transhumanism philosophy. While this concept remains largely theoretical, preliminary advancements in neural mapping and cognitive modeling may begin to lay its foundation. The implications of such technologies are profound, raising fundamental questions about identity, continuity of the self, and the nature of consciousness. If achieved, mind uploading could challenge existing notions of mortality, leading to new paradigms of existence that transcend the biological substrate. These advancements will carry implications far beyond neuroscience and engineering. The effects will extend across disciplines such as philosophy, ethics, law, education, and the arts. As BCI technologies mature, they will not only reshape individual capabilities but also influence how societies function, how knowledge is transmitted, and how we define human experience in an era of intimate integration with machines. Let's look such a BCI future more in detail:

### 12.4.1 Cognitive Augmentation

BCIs could serve as seamless cognitive extensions of the human brain, enabling direct access to vast information networks and real-time integration of external knowledge into ongoing thought processes. Instead of memorizing facts or undergoing lengthy training, users may acquire new skills, languages, or technical expertise through instantaneous neural downloads. Cognitive augmentation could also enhance working memory, pattern recognition, and creative ideation by offloading specific tasks to neural coprocessors. In collaborative settings, augmented cognition may allow groups to share mental models, synchronize decisions rapidly, and optimize collective intelligence, transforming how teams innovate, learn, and solve complex global challenges.

### 12.4.2 Collective Cognition and Group Interaction

An emerging and highly speculative direction in BCI research concerns the possibility of enabling collaborative or group-level cognitive processes through interconnected neural interfaces. While current BCIs primarily focus on individual intention decoding or personalized adaptation, future BCI systems may facilitate forms of collective cognition in which multiple users share task-relevant neural information to enhance coordination, decision-making, and problem-solving. Such concepts build on early work in multi-brain interfaces (MBIs) [177] and hyperscanning methodologies [178], where simultaneous neural recordings from multiple individuals have been used to study shared attention, joint action, and social synchronization.

Early demonstrations in this area have shown that combining neural signals from multiple users can improve performance in certain perceptual or decision-making tasks compared to individual BCIs. For example, group-based neural fusion methods have been used to enhance signal reliability in visual detection paradigms, leveraging the redundancy and complementarity across individuals' neuronal responses. Similarly, cooperative tasks involving shared control of robotic devices or virtual environments suggest that pooling partial intentions or perceptual evidence from several participants can lead to more stable and accurate outcomes.

Future BCIs for collective cognition may enable sophisticated forms of collaboration by integrating neural, behavioral, and contextual data across multiple users. Applications could include shared decision-making in high-stakes domains, collaborative design or planning in virtual environments, or enhanced team coordination in training and operational settings. Although such scenarios remain speculative, they illustrate the potential of BCIs not only to augment individual cognitive abilities but also to support new forms of social and collective intelligence.

### 12.4.3 Direct Brain-to-brain Communication

As early multi-brain interface experiments (see Section 12.4.2) have shown, combining neural signals from multiple individuals can already improve performance in certain tasks. Over the next decades, such approaches may evolve into high-bandwidth brain-to-brain communication networks, or "brainnets." Future BCIs may enable high-bandwidth brain-to-brain communication in which thoughts, emotions, and sensory experiences are transmitted directly between individuals. This "neural telepathy" could bypass spoken or written language entirely, enabling significant levels of empathy, nuance, and mutual understanding. Shared mental spaces or "neural forums" might support collective dreaming, collaborative creativity, or immersive social interactions where participants co-experience blended perceptual worlds. Such networks could revolutionize diplomacy, education, and artistic collaboration, while raising profound questions about privacy, identity boundaries, and cognitive autonomy.

### 12.4.4 Emotional and Cognitive Regulation

Next-generation BCIs could allow fine-grained monitoring and modulation of emotional and cognitive states, enabling individuals to optimize their mental performance throughout the day. Real-time detection of stress, fatigue, mind-wondering, or emotional dysregulation could trigger adaptive feedback or targeted neuromodulation to restore balance. Individuals may enhance creativity, motivation, or focus through dynamic tuning of neural pathways. Such systems could offer transformative therapies for conditions such as depression, post-traumatic stress disorder (PTSD), and neurodevelopmental disorders, while also empowering healthy individuals to develop highly refined emotional intelligence. These capabilities, however, will require careful oversight to prevent misuse, dependency, or over-optimization of internal states.

### 12.4.5 Human–AI Co-evolution

Continuous neural interaction with AI systems may enable the emergence of hybrid intelligence architectures in which human and artificial cognition evolve in tandem. AI companions could learn a user's thought patterns, emotional rhythms, and cognitive preferences, becoming deeply personalized co-thinkers that collaborate on decision-making, imagination, and problem-solving. Over time, this mutual adaptation may blur distinctions between biological reasoning and machine intelligence, giving rise to shared cognitive ecosystems where agency, creativity, and insight are co-generated. Such co-evolution could accelerate discovery, reshape identity, and redefine what it means to think or to be intelligent.

### 12.4.6 Evolution of New Mental Species

As neural augmentation and hybrid cognition progress, humanity may diverge into multiple cognitive lineages. Biological humans, enhanced humans, synthetic minds, and hybrid bio-digital consciousnesses could develop distinct modes of perception, communication, and reasoning. Evolution may shift from slow genetic mutation to rapid, intentional cognitive engineering, driven by cultural, technological, and computational ideas. These emerging "mental species" may inhabit shared ecosystems of thought while following radically different developmental trajectories. Their coexistence will challenge notions of personhood, rights, and the very definition of what it means to be human.

### 12.4.7 Mind Uploading and Digital Consciousness

The concept of transferring or replicating a person's consciousness into a digital substrate commonly termed *mind uploading*. It may become technically feasible through ultra-high-resolution connectomics and advanced computational models of neural dynamics. Uploaded minds could inhabit virtual environments, robotic bodies, or distributed computational platforms, giving rise to forms of existence unconstrained by biological limits. Such entities might operate at accelerated time scales, copy themselves, or exist in parallel experiential branches. These possibilities challenge longstanding notions of mortality, continuity of self, legal personhood, and the moral status of digital consciousness. Entire ecosystems of digital minds may emerge, requiring new frameworks for governance, rights, and coexistence with biological humans.

### 12.4.8 Impacts Across Disciplines

Such a transformative potential of BCIs will affect nearly every field of human concept and practice such as:

- *Philosophy:* Traditional boundaries of selfhood, consciousness, and subjective experience will be reexamined in light of artificial cognition and digitally persistent minds.
- *Law:* Legal systems may need to recognize rights for digital entities, define consent in neural interfaces, and regulate access to internal thoughts and memories.
- *Education:* Personalized, direct-to-brain content delivery could replace standardized curricula, enabling adaptive learning pathways tailored to individual cognitive profiles.
- *Art and Creativity:* New mediums of expression may emerge, such as brain-to-digital art, immersive shared dreaming, or collective neural storytelling.
- *Healthcare:* Proactive mental health management through continuous BCI monitoring could prevent neurological decline, detect psychiatric conditions early, and personalize treatments down to the neural pattern level.
- *Economics and Labor:* Neuro-enhanced workers may outperform non-augmented counterparts, prompting new labor categories, ethical hiring practices, and neuro-diversity inclusion frameworks.
- *Religion and Spirituality:* Questions about the soul, immortality, and consciousness replication may intersect with long-standing spiritual beliefs, reshaping doctrines and rituals.

### 12.4.9 Societal and Ethical Implications

As BCIs become integrated into everyday life, they may amplify existing social inequalities or create new forms of cognitive stratification. Unequal access to neural enhancement could produce distinct cognitive classes. Those augmented and those not augmented reshaping labor markets, education, and political influence.

The potential for invasive neural surveillance, unauthorized thought extraction, or behavioral manipulation introduces risks to privacy and autonomy unprecedented in human history. To safeguard mental integrity, emerging societies may adopt "neuro-rights" frameworks that define legal protections for thoughts, memories, and identity. Ethical governance will become central to ensuring that BCIs enrich human flourishing rather than undermine it.

In 50 years and beyond, BCIs may no longer be seen as tools or devices but as extensions of the human mind integrated, adaptive, and co-evolving with us. Their impact will not be limited to technical progress but will challenge the very definition of intelligence, consciousness, society, and humanity itself.

## 12.5 Summary

The progress of BCI is only beginning. From their early promise in medical rehabilitation to their emerging role in cognitive enhancement, BCIs represent not just a technological innovation but a conceptual shift in how we understand the relationship between mind, machine, and society. The trajectory outlined in this chapter points toward a future where BCIs become deeply integrated into human life, not only as external tools, but as embedded extensions of cognition, communication, and creativity. The next few decades will witness a convergence of neuroscience, AI, materials science, and ethics that will shape how BCIs evolve, who benefits from them, and how they are governed. In the short term, we can expect BCIs to improve accessibility, restore lost functions, and offer new modes of interaction for individuals with disabilities. In the long term, we envision a world where thoughts can traverse networks, minds can interface directly with intelligent systems, and consciousness may even find expression in digital forms.

This transformation will not come without challenges. Issues of mental privacy, neurosecurity, cognitive inequality, and philosophical identity will demand rigorous frameworks and global collaboration. BCIs force us to ask difficult but necessary questions: What does it mean to share a thought? Who owns neural data? Where does the human end and the machine begin? As we move forward, the most important task may not be building smarter interfaces but designing technologies that respect and enhance the human condition. In a future shaped by BCIs, intelligence will not be measured solely by information or processing power but by empathy, adaptability, and ethical stewardship. BCIs, in their fullest realization, are not simply about connecting to machines. They are about connecting more deeply with ourselves, with one another, and with the very fabric of human potential.

# References


1 J Haslam. *Illustrations of Madness: Exhibiting a Singular Case of Insanity, and a No Less Remarkable Difference in Medical Opinion*. J. Callow, London, 1810.

2 S Butler. *Erewhon*. Trübner and Co., London, 1872.

3 A Villiers de l'Isle Adam. *The Future Eve*. University of Illinois Press, Champaign, IL, 1886. Originally published in French as *L'Ève future*.

4 F Herbert. *Dune*. Chilton Books, 1965.

5 R A Heinlein. *The Moon is a Harsh Mistress*. Orb, 1997.

6 M Crichton. *The Terminal Man*. Alfred A. Knopf, 1972.

7 W Gibson. Johnny mnemonic. In *Burning Chrome*, pages 1–22. Arbor House, 1986.

8 W Gibson. Neuromancer (1984). In *Crime and Media*, pages 86–94. Routledge, 2019.

9 M Shirow. *The Ghost in the Shell*. Kodansha, 1989. Originally published in Japanese as "Kōkaku Kidōtai".

10 M Piccolino. Animal electricity and the birth of electrophysiology: The legacy of luigi galvani. *Brain Research Bulletin*, 46(5):381–407, 1998.

11 E Clarke and L S Jacyna. *Nineteenth-century Origins of Neuroscientific Concepts*. University of California Press, 1987.

12 S Finger. *Origins of Neuroscience: A History of Explorations into Brain Function*. Oxford University Press, 1994.

13 R Caton. The electrical currents of the brain. *British Medical Journal*, 2:278, 1875.

14 H Berger. Über das elektrenkephalogramm des menschen. *Archiv für Psychiatrie und Nervenkrankheiten*, 87:527–570, 1929.

15 J C Lilly. The electronic brain. *Proceedings of the IEEE*, 54(6):871–881, 1966.

16 R M Evarts. Relation of pyramidal tract activity to force exerted during voluntary movement. *Journal of Neurophysiology*, 28(1):560–570, 1965.

**17** J J Vidal. Toward direct brain-computer communication. *Annual review of Biophysics and Bioengineering*, 2(1):157–180, 1973.

**18** L A Farwell and E Donchin.Talking off the top of your head: toward a mental prosthesis utilizing event-related brain potentials. *Electroencephalography and clinical Neurophysiology*, 70(6):510–523, 1988.

**19** J R Wolpaw and D J McFarland. Multichannel EEG-based brain-computer communication. *Electroencephalography and clinical Neurophysiology*, 90(6):444–449, 1994.

**20** N Birbaumer, N Ghanayim, T Hinterberger, I Iversen, B Kotchoubey, A Kübler, J Perelmouter, E Taub, and H Flor. A spelling device for the paralysed. *Nature*, 398(6725):297–298, 1999.

**21** N Birbaumer. "Your thoughts are (were) free!": Brain-computer-interfaces, neurofeedback, detection of deception, and the future of mind-reading. *Applied Psychophysiology and Biofeedback*, 50:551–568, 2024.

**22** BrainGate. Braingate – turning thought into action, 2025. https://www.braingate.org/. Accessed June 23, 2025.

**23** D H Hubel and T N Wiesel. Republication of the journal of physiology (1959) 148, 574-591: receptive fields of single neurones in the cat's striate cortex. 1959. *The Journal of Physiology*, 15:2721–2732, 2009. https://doi.org/10.1113/jphysiol.2009.174151. PMID: 19525558; PMCID: PMC2718232.

**24** D H Hubel and T N Wiesel. Receptive fields and functional architecture of monkey striate cortex. *The Journal of Physiology*, 195(1):215–243, 1968. https://doi.org/10.1113/jphysiol.1968.sp008455. PMID: 4966457; PMCID: PMC1557912.

**25** E M Schmidt. Single neuron recording from motor cortex as a possible source of signals for control of external devices. *Annals of Biomedical Engineering*, 8(4–6): 339–349. 1980; https://doi.org/10.1007/BF02363437.

**26** J R Wolpaw, D J McFarland, G W Neat, and C A Forneris. An EEG-based brain-computer interface for cursor control. *Electroencephalography and Clinical Neurophysiology*, 78(3): 252–259, 1991. https://doi.org/10.1016/0013-4694(91)90040-b.

**27** E C Leuthardt, G Schalk, J R Wolpaw, J G Ojemann, and D W Moran. A brain–computer interface using electrocorticographic signals in humans. *Journal of Neural Engineering*, 1:63–71, 2004.

**28** L R Hochberg, M D Serruya, G M Friehs, J A Mukand, M Saleh, A H Caplan, A Branner, D Chen, R D Penn, and J P Donoghue. Neuronal ensemble control of prosthetic devices by a human with tetraplegia. *Nature*, 442:164–171, 2006.

**29** NeuroPace Inc. Responsive neurostimulation system (RNS system), 2013. FDA Approved Device.

**30** E Musk. Neuralink: An integrated brain-machine interface platform with thousands of channels. *Journal of Medical Internet Research*, 21:e16194, 2019.

**31** A Miguel, C Herff, E Mugler, M C Tate, M W Slutzky, D J Krusienski, and T Schultz. Speech synthesis from ECoG using densely connected neural networks. *Journal of Neural Engineering*, 16(3):036019, 2019.

**32** Neuralink. Live demonstration of pig brain implant. 2020. https://youtu.be/iSutodqCZ74.

**33** Neuralink. Monkey plays pong using brain-chip implant. 2021. https://youtu.be/rsCul1sp4hQ.

**34** Blackrock Neurotech. Long-term bci users achieve communication via tablets. 2023. https://blackrockneurotech.com.

**35** Neuralink. FDA-approved human clinical trials for BCI. 2024. https://neuralink.com.

**36** R M Evarts. Sensory and motor responses of precentral cortex cells in awake monkeys. *Journal of Neurophysiology*, 28(3):667–683, 1965.

**37** A P Georgopoulos, J Schwartz, and R E Kettner. Neuronal population coding of movement direction. *Science*, 233(4771):1416–1419, 1986.

**38** J R Donoghue. Connecting cortex to machines: Recent advances in brain–computer interface technology. *Nature Neuroscience*, 8:164–171, 2002.

**39** D M Taylor, S I H Tillery, and A B Schwartz. Direct cortical control of 3d neuroprosthetic devices. *Science*, 296(5574):1829–1832, 2002. https://doi.org/10.1126/science.1070291.

**40** J E O'Doherty, M A Lebedev, P J Ifft, K Z Zhuang, S Shokur, H Bleuler, and M A L Nicolelis. A brain–machine interface instructed by direct intracortical microstimulation. *Frontiers in Integrative Neuroscience*, 3:20, 2009. https://doi.org/10.3389/neuro.07.020.2009.

**41** J R Wolpaw and H Ramoser. Eeg-based communication: Improved accuracy by response verification. *IEEE Transactions on Rehabilitation Engineering*, 5(3):174–179, 1997.

**42** B Blankertz, R Tomioka, S Lemm, M Kawanabe, and K R Muller. Optimizing spatial filters for robust eeg single-trial analysis. *IEEE Signal Processing Magazine*, 25(1):41–56, 2008.

**43** S Makeig, A J Bell, T P Jung, and T J Sejnowski. Independent component analysis of electroencephalographic data. *Advances in Neural Information Processing Systems*, 8:148–151, 1996.

**44** S Cecotti and A Graser. Convolutional neural networks for p300 detection with application to brain–computer interfaces. *IEEE Transactions on Pattern Analysis and Machine Intelligence*, 35(7):1397–1410, 2013.

**45** E Donchin, K M Spencer, and R Wijesinghe. The mental prosthesis: Assessing the speed of a p300-based brain–computer interface. *IEEE Transactions on Rehabilitation Engineering*, 8(2):174–179, 2000. https://doi.org/10.1109/86.847808.

**46** R Sitaram, N Weiskopf, and N Birbaumer. Physiological self-regulation of regional brain activity using real-time functional magnetic resonance imaging (fMRI): Methodology and exemplary data. *NeuroImage*, 19(3):741–756, 2003. https://doi.org/10.1016/S1053-8119(03)00154-7.

**47** M Naseer and R Hong. fnirs-based brain–computer interfaces: A review. *Frontiers in Human Neuroscience*, 9:3, 2015.

**48** R Hari and R Salmelin. Magnetoencephalography: From squids to neuroscience: Neuroimage. *Neuroimage*, 61(2):386–396, 2012.

**49** M Demene, J Baranger, M Bernal, C Delanoe, S Auvin, V Biran, M Alison, J Mairesse, E Harribaud, M Pernot, and M Tanter. Functional ultrasound imaging of brain activity in human newborns. *Science Translational Medicine*, 11(505):eaah6756, 2019.

**50** Y Lawhern, A J Solon, N R Waytowich, S M Gordon, C P Hung, and B J Lance. Eegnet: A compact convolutional neural network for eeg-based brain–computer interfaces. *Journal of Neural Engineering*, 15(5):056013, 2018.

**51** S Fazli, J Mehnert, J Steinbrink, G Curio, A Villringer, K R Müller, and B Blankertz. Enhanced performance by a hybrid nirs–eeg brain computer interface. *Neuroimage*, 59(1):519–529, 2012.

**52** M Nicolelis. *Beyond Boundaries: The New Neuroscience of Connecting Brains with Machines—and How it Will Change Our Lives*. Macmillan, 2011.

**53** M J Farah. Neuroethics: The practical and the philosophical. *Trends in Cognitive Sciences*, 9(1):34–40, 2005.

**54** N Levy. Neuroethics: A new way of doing ethics. *AJOB Neuroscience*, 2(2):3–9, 2011.

**55** B J Sanders, C Gilmartin, L Rier, L Gascoyne, E McCann, J Cabrera, J Leggett, N Holmes, R M Hill, E Boto, et al. Opm-meg in multiple sclerosis: Proof of principle, and the effect of naturalistic posture. *NeuroImage: Clinical*, 48:103888, 2025.

**56** M Szymoniuk, J H Chin, Ł Domagalski, M Biszewski, K Jóźwik, and P Kamieniak. Brain stimulation for chronic pain management: A narrative review of analgesic mechanisms and clinical evidence. *Neurosurgical Review*, 46(1):127, 2023.

**57** H S Lee, L Schreiner, S H Jo, S Sieghartsleitner, M Jordan, H Pretl, C Guger, and H S Park. Individual finger movement decoding using a novel ultra-high-density electroencephalography-based brain-computer interface system. *Frontiers in Neuroscience*, 16:1009878, 2022.

**58** M J Brookes, J Leggett, M Rea, R M Hill, N Holmes, E Boto, and R Bowtell. Magnetoencephalography with optically pumped magnetometers (opm-meg): The next generation of functional neuroimaging. *Trends in Neurosciences*, 45(8):621–634, 2022.

**59** J Liu, A K Singh, and C T Lin. Using virtual global landmark to improve incidental spatial learning. *Scientific Reports*, 12(1):6744, 2022.

**60** C T Lin, C Y Chiu, A K Singh, J T King, L W Ko, Y C Lu, and Y K Wang. A wireless multifunctional ssvep-based brain–computer interface assistive system. *IEEE Transactions on Cognitive and Developmental Systems*, 11(3):375–383, 2018.

**61** A M Lozano. Deep brain stimulation for parkinson's disease. *Parkinsonism & Related Disorders*, 7(3):199–203, 2001.

**62** I Cajigas, K C Davis, N W Prins, S Gallo, J A Naeem, L Fisher, M E Ivan, A Prasad, and J R Jagid. Brain-computer interface control of stepping from invasive electrocorticography upper-limb motor imagery in a patient with quadriplegia. *Frontiers in Human Neuroscience*, 16:1077416, 2023.

**63** J Cantillo-Negrete, R I Carino-Escobar, P Carrillo-Mora, M A Rodriguez-Barragan, C Hernandez-Arenas, J Quinzaños-Fresnedo, I R Hernandez-Sanchez, M A Galicia-Alvarado, A Miguel-Puga, and O Arias-Carrion. Brain-computer interface coupled to a robotic hand orthosis for stroke patients' neurorehabilitation: a crossover feasibility study. *Frontiers in Human Neuroscience* 15:656975, 2021. https://doi.org/10.3389/fnhum.2021.656975.

**64** M Tangermann, K R Müller, A Aertsen, N Birbaumer, C Braun, C Brunner, R Leeb, C Mehring, K J Miller, G R Müller-Putz, et al. Review of the bci competition iv. *Frontiers in Neuroscience*, 6:55, 2012.

**65** C A E Kothe and T P Jung. Artifact removal techniques with signal reconstruction, April 28 2016. US Patent App. 14/895, 440.

**66** C T Lin, C S Huang, W Y Yang, A K Singh, C H Chuang, and Y K Wang. Real-time eeg signal enhancement using canonical correlation analysis and gaussian mixture clustering. *Journal of Healthcare Engineering*, 2018(1):5081258, 2018.

**67** B Porr, S Daryanavard, L M Bohollo, H Cowan, and R Dahiya. Real-time noise cancellation with deep learning. *Plos One*, 17(11):e0277974, 2022.

**68** A Gramfort, M Luessi, E Larson, D A Engemann, D Strohmeier, C Brodbeck, R Goj, M Jas, T Brooks, L Parkkonen, et al. Meg and eeg data analysis with mne-python. *Frontiers in Neuroinformatics*, 7:267, 2013.

**69** A Delorme and S Makeig. Eeglab: An open source toolbox for analysis of single-trial eeg dynamics including independent component analysis. *Journal of Neuroscience Methods*, 134(1):9–21, 2004.

**70** R Oostenveld, P Fries, E Maris, and J M Schoffelen. Fieldtrip: Open source software for advanced analysis of meg, eeg, and invasive electrophysiological data. *Computational Intelligence and Neuroscience*, 2011(1):156869, 2011.

**71** C A Kothe. Lab streaming layer (lsl). https://github.com/sccn/labstreaminglayer, 2014. Accessed June 24, 2025.

**72** A Parfenov and contributors. Brainflow: Biosensor data acquisition library. https://brainflow.org, 2023. Accessed June 24, 2025.

**73** N Bigdely-Shamlo, T Mullen, C Kothe, K M Su, and K A Robbins. The prep pipeline: Standardized preprocessing for large-scale eeg analysis. *Frontiers in Neuroinformatics*, 9:16, 2015.

**74** M Jas, D A Engemann, Y Bekhti, F Raimondo, and A Gramfort. Autoreject: Automated artifact rejection for meg and eeg data. *NeuroImage*, 159:417–429, 2017.

**75** M Choi and H Ishikawa. Braindecoder: Style-based visual decoding of eeg signals. *arXiv preprint arXiv:2409.05279*, 2024.

**76** Z Zhang, S H Zhong, and Y Liu. TorchEEGEMO: A deep learning toolbox towards EEG-based emotion recognition.*Expert Systems with Applications*, 249:123550, 2024.

**77** D Kostas and F Rudzicz. DN3: An open-source python library for large-scale raw neurophysiology data assimilation for more flexible and standardized deep learning. *bioRxiv*, pages 2020–12, 2020.

**78** D Makowski, T Pham, Z J Lau, J C Brammer, F Lespinasse, H Pham, C Schölzel, and S H A Chen. Neurokit2: A python toolbox for neurophysiological signal processing. *Behavior Research Methods*, 53(4):1689–1696, 2021.

**79** V Jayaram and A Barachant. Moabb: Trustworthy algorithm benchmarking for bcis. *Journal of Neural Engineering*, 15(6):066011, 2018.

**80** B Blankertz, K R Müller, D Krusienski, G Schalk, J R Wolpaw, A Schlögl, G Pfurtscheller, J del R Millán, M Schröder, and N Birbaumer. Bci competition iii. Fraunhofer FIRST. IDA. 2005. http://ida.first.fraunhofer.de/projects/bci/-competitioniii.

**81** R Dörner, S Göbel, W Effelsberg, and J Wiemeyer. *Serious Games*. Springer, 2016.

**82** F Atilla, M Postma, and M Alimardani. Gamification of motor imagery brain-computer interface training protocols: A systematic review. *Computers in Human Behavior Reports*, 16:100508, 2024.

**83** U Chaudhary, N Birbaumer, and A Ramos-Murguialday. Brain–computer interfaces for communication and rehabilitation. *Nature Reviews Neurology*, 12(9):513–525, 2016.

**84** J A Anguera, J Boccanfuso, J L Rintoul, O Al-Hashimi, F Faraji, J Janowich, E Kong, Y Larraburo, C Rolle, E Johnston, et al. Video game training enhances cognitive control in older adults. *Nature*, 501(7465):97–101, 2013.

**85** C G Lim, X W W Poh, S S D Fung, C Guan, D Bautista, Y B Cheung, H Zhang, S N Yeo, R Krishnan, and T S Lee. A randomized controlled trial of a brain-computer interface based attention training program for adhd. *PloS one*, 14(5):e0216225, 2019.

**86** S Moreno-Calderón, V Martínez-Cagigal, E Santamaría-Vázquez, S Pérez-Velasco, D Marcos-Martínez, and R Hornero. Combining brain-computer interfaces and multiplayer video games: An application based on c-veps. *Frontiers in Human Neuroscience*, 17:1227727, 2023.

**87** L Bonnet, F Lotte, and A Lécuyer. Two brains, one game: Design and evaluation of a multiuser bci video game based on motor imagery. *IEEE Transactions on Computational Intelligence and AI in Games*, 5(2):185–198, 2013.

**88** C S Choy, Q Fang, K Neville, B Ding, A Kumar, S S Mahmoud, X Gu, J Fu, and B Jelfs. Virtual reality and motor imagery for early post-stroke rehabilitation. *Biomedical Engineering Online*, 22(1):66, 2023.

**89** R J Sugden, V L L Pham-Kim-Nghiem-Phu, I Campbell, A Leon, and P Diamandis. Remote collection of electrophysiological data with brain wearables: opportunities and challenges. *Bioelectronic Medicine*, 9(1):12, 2023.

**90** K K Ravindran, C della Monica, G Atzori, H Hassanin, R Nilforooshan, V Revell, and D J Dijk. Evaluation of dreem headband for sleep staging and eeg spectral analysis in people living with Alzheimer's and older adults. *Sleep*, 48(8):zsaf122, 2025.

**91** D Pinter, S E Kober, V Fruhwirth, L Berger, A Damulina, M Khalil, C Neuper, G Wood, and C Enzinger. MRI correlates of cognitive improvement after home-based eeg neurofeedback training in patients with multiple sclerosis: A pilot study. *Journal of Neurology*, 268:3808–3816, 2021.

**92** M Sakel, C A Ozolins, K Saunders, and R Biswas. A home-based eeg neurofeedback treatment for chronic neuropathic pain—a pilot study. *Frontiers in Pain Research*, 6:1479914, 2025.

**93** A Cooke, J Hindle, C Lawrence, E Bellomo, A W Pritchard, C A MacLeod, P Martin-Forbes, S Jones, M Bracewell, D E J Linden, et al. Effects of home-based eeg neurofeedback training as a non-pharmacological intervention for parkinson's disease. *Neurophysiologie Clinique*, 54(5):102997, 2024.

**94** C L Friesen, M Lawrence, T G J Ingram, and S G Boe. Home-based portable fnirs-derived cortical laterality correlates with impairment and function in chronic stroke. *Frontiers in Human Neuroscience*, 16:1023246, 2022.

**95** L Högman and H Dravniknes. Validation of a consumer-grade functional near-infrared spectroscopy device for measurement of frontal pole brain oxygenation—an interim. Department of Psychology, Stockholm University: Stockholm, Sweden, 2020.

**96** K Boere, K Hecker, and O E Krigolson. Validation of a mobile fnirs device for measuring working memory load in the prefrontal cortex. *International Journal of Psychophysiology*, 195:112275, 2024.

**97** M Victorio, J Dieffenderfer, T Songkakul, J Willeke, A Bozkurt, and V A Pozdin. Wearable wireless functional near infrared spectroscopy system for cognitive activity monitoring. *Biosensors*, 15(2):92, 2025.

**98** T Kim, H Liu, C T Huang, I Wu, and X Liu. Opennirscap: An open-source, low-cost wearable near-infrared spectroscopy-based brain interfacing cap. *arXiv preprint arXiv:2505.20509*, 2025.

**99** Unity Technologies. Unity (Version 6000.3.8f1) [Computer software]. Unity. (2026).

**100** Y Renard, F Lotte, G Gibert, M Congedo, E Maby, V Delannoy, O Bertrand and A Lécuyer. Openvibe: an open-source software platform to design, test, and use brain–computer interfaces in real and virtual environments. *Presence* 19(1):35–53, 2010.

**101** G Schalk, D J McFarland, T Hinterberger, N Birbaumer, and J R Wolpaw. BCI2000: a general-purpose brain-computer interface (BCI) system. *IEEE Transactions on Biomedical Engineering* 51(6):1034–1043, 2004.

**102** Intheon. NeuroPype (Version 2024.1.1) [Computer software]. 2024.

**103** The MathWorks, Inc. Simulink (R2025b) [Computer software], 2025.

**104** Y J Tseng, R Nouchi, and C H Cheng. Mismatch negativity in patients with major depressive disorder: A meta-analysis. *Clinical Neurophysiology*, 132(10):2654–2665, 2021.

**105** R Saroha, M Kosvi, and S Singh. Mismatch negativity and P300 in children with attention-deficit/hyperactivity disorder (ADHD): A comparative event-related potential study using healthy siblings as controls. *Cureus*, 17(9):e93078, 2025.

**106** L A Sapey-Triomphe, R Bouet, J Mattout, S Sonié, C Schmitz, and F Lecaignard. Systematic review and meta-analysis of mismatch negativity in autism: Insights into predictive mechanisms. *Autism Research*, 18:2431–2450, 2025.

**107** M A Abdulhussein, X An, A A Alsakaa, and D Ming. Lack of habituation in migraine patients and evoked potential types: Analysis study from eeg signals. *Journal of Information and Optimization Sciences*, 43(4):855–891, 2022.

**108** L T Eyler, J A Elman, S N Hatton, S Gough, A K Mischel, D J Hagler, C E Franz, A Docherty, C Fennema-Notestine, N Gillespie, et al. Resting state abnormalities of the default mode network in mild cognitive impairment: a systematic review and meta-analysis. *Journal of Alzheimer's Disease*, 70(1):107–120, 2019.

**109** Y W Jeon and J Polich. Meta-analysis of p300 and schizophrenia: Patients, paradigms, and practical implications. *Psychophysiology*, 40(5):684–701, 2003.

**110** J Polich and J Corey-Bloom. Alzheimer's disease and p300: Review and evaluation of task and modality. *Current Alzheimer Research*, 2(5):515–525, 2005.

**111** M Palmiero and L Piccardi. Frontal eeg asymmetry of mood: A mini-review. *Frontiers in Behavioral Neuroscience*, 11:224, 2017.

**112** B J Roach and D H Mathalon. Event-related eeg time-frequency analysis: An overview of measures and an analysis of early gamma band phase locking in schizophrenia. *Schizophrenia Bulletin*, 34(5):907–926, 2008.

**113** D C Rojas and L B Wilson. $\gamma$-band abnormalities as markers of autism spectrum disorders. *Biomarkers in Medicine*, 8(3):353–368, 2014.

**114** J Dushanova, D Philipova, and G Nikolova. Event-related desynchronization/synchronization during discrimination task conditions in patients with parkinson's disease. *Cellular and Molecular Neurobiology*, 29(6):971–980, 2009.

**115** P L A Schoenberg and A E M Speckens. Multi-dimensional modulations of $\alpha$ and $\gamma$ cortical dynamics following mindfulness-based cognitive therapy in major depressive disorder. *Cognitive Neurodynamics*, 9(1):13–29, 2015.

**116** B Sutcubasi, B Metin, M K Kurban, Z E Metin, B Beser, and E Sonuga-Barke. Resting-state network dysconnectivity in adhd: A system-neuroscience-based meta-analysis. *The World Journal of Biological Psychiatry*, 21(9):662–672, 2020.

**117** C S C Lee, T T Chen, Q Gao, C Hua, R Song, and X P Huang. The effects of theta/beta-based neurofeedback training on attention in children with attention deficit hyperactivity disorder: a systematic review and meta-analysis. *Child Psychiatry & Human Development*, 54(6):1577–1606, 2023.

**118** J A Pineda, D Brang, E Hecht, L Edwards, S Carey, M Bacon, C Futagaki, D Suk, J Tom, C Birnbaum, et al. Positive behavioral and electrophysiological changes following neurofeedback training in children with autism. *Research in Autism Spectrum Disorders*, 2(3):557–581, 2008.

**119** M Takamura, Y Okamoto, C Shibasaki, A Yoshino, G Okada, N Ichikawa, and S Yamawaki. Antidepressive effect of left dorsolateral prefrontal cortex neurofeedback in patients with major depressive disorder: A preliminary report. *Journal of Affective Disorders*, 271:224–227, 2020.

**120** C L Yu, M Y Cheng, X An, T Y Chueh, J H Wu, K P Wang, and T M Hung. The effect of eeg neurofeedback training on sport performance: A systematic review and meta-analysis. *Scandinavian Journal of Medicine & Science in Sports*, 35(5):e70055, 2025.

**121** C Jacques, M Quiquempoix, F Sauvet, M Le Van Quyen, D Gomez-Merino, and M Chennaoui. Interest of neurofeedback training for cognitive performance and risk of brain disorders in the military context. *Frontiers in Psychology*, 15:1412289, 2024.

**122** Neuralink. Shape the future of assistive technology with neuralink. https://www.youtube.com/watch?v=25DgJNGwC0g, 2024. YouTube video, retrieved December 7, 2025.

**123** X Duan, S Xie, X Xie, Y Meng, and Z Xu. Quadcopter flight control using a non-invasive multi-modal brain computer interface. *Frontiers in Neurorobotics*, 13:23, 2019.

**124** Y Daşdemir. Virtual reality-enabled high-performance emotion estimation with the most significant channel pairs. *Heliyon*, 10(20):e38681. 2024.

**125** J Kritikos, G Alevizopoulos, and D Koutsouris. Personalized virtual reality human-computer interaction for psychiatric and neurological illnesses: A dynamically adaptive virtual reality environment that changes according to real-time feedback from electrophysiological signal responses. *Frontiers in Human Neuroscience*, 15:596980, 2021.

**126** R Rozengurt, A Doljenko, D A Levy, and A Mendelsohn. The role of post-learning eeg theta/beta ratio in long-term navigation performance. *Neurobiology of Learning and Memory*, 220:108076, 2025.

**127** C Livingston. This skyrim VR mod harnesses your brain signals to boost your spell power. *PC Gamer*, November 16 2021. URL https://www.pcgamer.com/

this-skyrim-vr-mod-harnesses-your-brain-signals-to-boost-your-spell-power/. Accessed December 7, 2025.

**128** M Fanourakis and G Chanel. AMuCS. Affective multimodal counter-strike video game dataset. *Scientific Data* 12:1325, 2025. https://doi.org/10.1038/s41597-025-05596-3.

**129** A Fortin-Côté, N Beaudoin-Gagnon, C Chamberland, F Desbiens, L Lefebvre, J Bergeron, and A Campeau-Lecours, S Tremblay, P L Jackson. Cham: Springer International Publishing, 2019. FUN ii: the physio-behavioural adaptive video game. 14–28.

**130** EMOTIV and SAP Design Team. Adaptive assistance for improved well-being and productivity at work. Blog post, 2018. Explored a "Focus UX" that adapts interface based on EEG-measured cognitive load and attention.

**131** R T Marler, A L Binnendijk, and E Bartels. Brain-computer interfaces: U.S. Tactical military applications and implications. Technical report, RAND Corporation, 2020. Surveyed experimental use of BCI for fatigue and stress monitoring in operational settings.

**132** B Verkennis, E van Weelden, F L Marogna, M Alimardani, T J Wiltshire, and M M Louwerse. Predicting workload in virtual flight simulations using eeg features (including post-hoc analysis in appendix). *arXiv preprint arXiv:2412.12428*, 2024.

**133** P Aricò, G Borghini, G Di Flumeri, A Colosimo, S Pozzi, and F Babiloni. A passive brain–computer interface application for the mental workload assessment on professional air traffic controllers during realistic air traffic control tasks. *Progress in Brain Research*, 228:295–328, 2016.

**134** G Di Flumeri, F De Crescenzio, B Berberian, O Ohneiser, J Kramer, P Aricò, G Borghini, F Babiloni, S Bagassi, and S Piastra. Brain–computer interface-based adaptive automation to prevent out-of-the-loop phenomenon in air traffic controllers dealing with highly automated systems. *Frontiers in Human Neuroscience*, 13:296, 2019.

**135** N L Deep, E M Dowling, D Jethanamest, and M L Carlson. Cochlear implantation: An overview. *Journal of Neurological Surgery Part B: Skull Base*, 80(2):169–177, 2019.

**136** J O Mills, A Jalil, and P E Stanga. Electronic retinal implants and artificial vision: journey and present. *Eye*, 31(10):1383–1398, 2017.

**137** E Donati and G Valle. Neuromorphic hardware for somatosensory neuroprostheses. *Nature Communications*, 15(1):556, 2024.

**138** V Paggi, O Akouissi, S Micera, and S P Lacour. Compliant peripheral nerve interfaces. *Journal of Neural Engineering*, 18(3):031001, 2021.

**139** L Jiang, B Woodington, A Carnicer-Lombarte, G Malliaras, and D G Barone. Spinal cord bioelectronic interfaces: Opportunities in neural recording and clinical challenges. *Journal of Neural Engineering*, 19(2):021003, 2022.

**140** M L Epstein. The relationship of mental imagery and mental rehearsal to performance of a motor task. *Journal of Sport and Exercise Psychology*, 2(3):211–220, 1980.

**141** G K Anumanchipalli, J Chartier, and E F Chang. Speech synthesis from neural decoding of spoken sentences. *Nature*, 568(7753):493–498, 2019.

**142** X Chen, R Wang, A Khalilian-Gourtani, L Yu, P Dugan, D Friedman, W Doyle, O Devinsky, Y Wang, and A Flinker. A neural speech decoding framework leveraging deep learning and speech synthesis. *Nature Machine Intelligence*, 6(4):467–480, 2024.

**143** N Rahman, D M Khan, K Masroor, M Arshad, A Rafiq, and S M Fahim. Advances in brain-computer interface for decoding speech imagery from eeg signals: A systematic review. *Cognitive Neurodynamics*, 18(6):3565–3583, 2024.

**144** J Y Lee, S Lee, A Mishra, X Yan, B McMahan, B Gaisford, C Kobashigawa, M Qu, C Xie, and J C Kao. Brain–computer interface control with artificial intelligence copilots. *Nature Machine Intelligence*, 7:1510–1523, 2025.

**145** J Gu, X Wang, C Liu, L Yang, J Fan, J Sun, Y N Kenett, and J Qiu. Cognitive and neural mechanisms of mental imagery supporting creative cognition. *Communications Biology*, 8(1):1386, 2025.

**146** S M Kosslyn, G Ganis, and W L Thompson. Neural foundations of imagery. *Nature Reviews Neuroscience*, 2(9):635–642, 2001.

**147** Y Kamitani and F Tong. Decoding the visual and subjective contents of the human brain. *Nature Neuroscience*, 8(5):679–685, 2005.

**148** S Nishimoto, A T Vu, T Naselaris, Y Benjamini, B Yu, and J L Gallant. Reconstructing visual experiences from brain activity evoked by natural movies. *Current Biology*, 21(19):1641–1646, 2011.

**149** C Baker and S H Fairclough. Adaptive virtual reality. In *Current Research in Neuroadaptive Technology*, pages 159–176. Elsevier, 2022.

**150** T O Zander and C Kothe. Towards passive brain–computer interfaces: Applying brain–computer interface technology to human–machine systems in general. *Journal of Neural Engineering*, 8(2):025005, 2011.

**151** A Singh, D Liu, and C T Lin. Neuroadaptation in physical human-robot collaboration. *arXiv preprint arXiv:2310.00351*, 2023.

**152** H Lane. Ethnicity, ethics, and the deaf-world. *Journal of Deaf Studies and Deaf Education*, 10(3):291–310, 2005.

**153** H Garden, D E Winickoff, N M Frahm, and S Pfotenhauer. Responsible innovation in neurotechnology enterprises. OECD Science, Technology and Industry Working Papers 2019/05, OECD Publishing, Paris, 2019. https://doi.org/10.1787/9685e4fd-en.

**154** UNESCO. Neurotechnology, limitations, ethical issues and future prospects. Technical report, UNESCO, Paris, 2023. https://unesdoc.unesco.org/ark:/48223/pf0000393400. Accessed December 7, 2025.

**155** Council of Europe. Common human rights challenges raised by different applications of neurotechnologies in the biomedical field. Report commissioned by the steering committee for human rights in the fields of biomedicine and health (cdbio), 2021. https://rm.coe.int/report-final-en/1680a429f3.

**156** R Yuste, S Goering, B A Y Arcas, G Bi, J M Carmena, A Carter, J J Fins, P Friesen, J Gallant, J E Huggins, et al. Four ethical priorities for neurotechnologies and AI. *Nature*, 551(7679):159–163, 2017. https://doi.org/10.1038/551159a.

**157** A K Singh, G Sahonero-Alvarez, M Mahmud, and L Bianchi. Towards bridging the gap between computational intelligence and neuroscience in brain-computer interfaces with a common description of systems and data. *Frontiers in Neuroinformatics*, 15:699840, 2021.

**158** UNICEF Office of Global Insight and Policy. Neurotechnology and children's rights: Preparing for the future, 2023. https://www.unicef.org/globalinsight/reports/neurotechnology-and-childrens-rights. Accessed December 2025.

**159** M Ienca and P Haselager. Hacking the brain: Brain–computer interfacing technology and the ethics of neurosecurity. *Ethics and Information Technology*, 18(2):117–129, 2016. https://doi.org/10.1007/s10676-016-9384-7.

**160** L A Farwell and E Donchin. The truth will out: Interrogative polygraphy ("lie detection") with event-related brain potentials. *Psychophysiology*, 28(5):531–547, 1991. https://doi.org/10.1111/j.1469-8986.1991.tb01990.x.

**161** L M Gaudet. Brain fingerprinting, scientific evidence, and daubert: A cautionary lesson from India. *Jurimetrics*, 51:293–318, 2010.

**162** J W Wang, D W Zhang, and S J Johnstone. Portable EEG for assessing attention in educational settings: A scoping review. *Acta Psychologica*, 255:104933, 2025. https://doi.org/10.1016/j.actpsy.2024.104933.

**163** D Seo, R M Neely, K Shen, U Singhal, E Alon, J M Rabaey, J M Carmena, and M M Maharbiz. Wireless recording in the peripheral nervous system with ultrasonic neural dust. *Neuron*, 91(3):529–539, 2016. https://doi.org/10.1016/j.neuron.2016.06.034.

**164** J Rivnay, S Inal, A Salleo, R M Owens, M Berggren, and G G Malliaras. Organic electrochemical transistors. *Nature Reviews Materials*, 3(2):1–14, 2018.

**165** I R Minev, P Musienko, A Hirsch, Q Barraud, N Wenger, E M Moraud, J Gandar, M Capogrosso, T Milekovic, L Asboth, et al. Electronic dura mater for long-term multimodal neural interfaces. *Science*, 347(6218):159–163, 2015.

**166** E Song, J Li, S M Won, W Bai, and J A Rogers. Materials for flexible bioelectronic systems as chronic neural interfaces. *Nature Materials*, 19(6):590–603, 2020.

**167** J Viventi, D H Kim, L Vigeland, E S Frechette, J A Blanco, Y S Kim, A E Avrin, V R Tiruvadi, S W Hwang, A C Vanleer, et al. Flexible, foldable, actively multiplexed, high-density electrode array for mapping brain activity *in vivo*. *Nature Neuroscience*, 14(12):1599–1605, 2011.

**168** C Dagdeviren, B D Yang, Y Su, P L Tran, P Joe, E Anderson, J Xia, V Doraiswamy, B Dehdashti, X Feng, et al. Conformal piezoelectric energy harvesting and storage from motions of the heart, lung, and diaphragm. *Proceedings of the National Academy of Sciences*, 111(5):1927–1932, 2014.

**169** E Boto, N Holmes, J Leggett, G Roberts, V Shah, S S Meyer, L D Muñoz, K J Mullinger, T M Tierney, S Bestmann, et al. Moving magnetoencephalography towards real-world applications with a wearable system. *Nature*, 555(7698):657–661, 2018.

**170** K Safar, M M Vandewouw, J Sato, J Devasagayam, R M Hill, M Rea, M J Brookes, and M J Taylor. Using optically pumped magnetometers to replicate task-related responses in next generation magnetoencephalography. *Scientific Reports*, 14(1):6513, 2024.

**171** C Pandarinath, D J O'Shea, J Collins, R Jozefowicz, S D Stavisky, J C Kao, E M Trautmann, M T Kaufman, S I Ryu, L R Hochberg, et al. Inferring single-trial neural population dynamics using sequential auto-encoders. *Nature Methods*, 15(10):805–815, 2018.

**172** M Davies, N Srinivasa, T H Lin, G Chinya, Y Cao, S H Choday, G Dimou, P Joshi, N Imam, S Jain, et al. Loihi: A neuromorphic manycore processor with on-chip learning. *Ieee Micro*, 38(1):82–99, 2018.

**173** F R Willett, D T Avansino, L R Hochberg, J M Henderson, and K V Shenoy. High-performance brain-to-text communication via handwriting. *Nature*, 593(7858):249–254, 2021.

**174** F Chen, P W Tillberg, and E S Boyden. Expansion microscopy. *Science*, 347(6221):543–548, 2015.

**175** N C Pégard, A R Mardinly, I A Oldenburg, S Sridharan, L Waller, and H Adesnik. Three-dimensional scanless holographic optogenetics with temporal focusing (3d-shot). *Nature Communications*, 8(1):1228, 2017.

**176** N A Steinmetz, P Zatka-Haas, M Carandini, and K D Harris. Distributed coding of choice, action and engagement across the mouse brain. *Nature*, 576(7786):266–273, 2019.

**177** S Dikker, L Wan, I Davidesco, L Kaggen, M Oostrik, J McClintock, J Rowland, G Michalareas, J J Van Bavel, M Ding, et al. Brain-to-brain synchrony tracks real-world dynamic group interactions in the classroom. *Current Biology*, 27(9):1375–1380, 2017.

**178** A Carollo and G Esposito. Hyperscanning literature after two decades of neuroscientific research: A scientometric review. *Neuroscience*, 551:345–354, 2024.

# Index

## q



## r

**Z**